Mental Health Across the Lifespan

Guest Editors

PATRICIA B. HOWARD, PhD, RN, CNAA, FAAN
PEGGY EL-MALLAKH, PhD, RN

NURSING CLINICS OF NORTH AMERICA

www.nursing.theclinics.com

Consulting Editor
SUZANNE S. PREVOST, RN, PhD, COI

December 2010 • Volume 45 • Number 4

SAUNDERS an imprint of ELSEVIER, Inc.

W.B. SAUNDERS COMPANY

A Division of Elsevier Inc.

1600 John F. Kennedy Blvd., Suite 1800 ● Philadelphia, PA 19103-2899

http://www.theclinics.com

NURSING CLINICS OF NORTH AMERICA Volume 45, Number 4
December 2010 ISSN 0029-6465, ISBN-13: 978-1-4377-2394-6

Editor: Katie Hartner
Developmental Editor: Donald Mumford

Nursing Clinics of North America (ISSN 0029-6465) is published quarterly by Elsevier Inc., 360 Park Avenue South, New York, NY 10010-1710. Months of issue are March, June, September, and December. Periodicals postage paid at New York, NY and additional mailing offices. Subscription price per year is, $135.00 (US individuals), $343.00 (US institutions), $244.00 (international individuals), $419.00 (international institutions), $197.00 (Canadian individuals), $419.00 (Canadian institutions), $74.00 (US students), and $121.00 (international students). To receive student/resident rate, orders must be accompanied by name of affiliated institution, date of term, and the signature of program/residency coordinator on institution letterhead. Orders will be billed at individual rate until proof of status is received. Foreign air speed delivery is included in all *Clinics* subscription prices. All prices are subject to change without notice. **POSTMASTER:** Send address changes to *Nursing Clinics*, Elsevier Health Sciences Division, Subscription Customer Service, 3251 Riverport Lane, Maryland Heights, MO 63043. **Customer Service: Telephone: 1-800-654-2452** (U.S. and Canada); **1-314-447-8871 (outside U.S. and Canada). Fax: 1-314-447-8029.** E-mail: journalscustomerservice-usa@elsevier.com (for print support) and **journalsonlinesupport-usa@elsevier.com** (for online support).

Nursing Clinics of North America is covered in *EMBASE/Excerpta Medica, MEDLINE/PubMed (Index Medicus), Social Sciences Citation Index, Current Contents, ASCA, Cumulative Index to Nursing, RNdex Top 100,* and Allied Health Literature and International Nursing Index (INI).

Printed and bound by CPI Group (UK) Ltd, Croydon, CR0 4YY

Transferred to Digital Print 2011

Contributors

CONSULTING EDITOR

SUZANNE S. PREVOST, PhD, RN, COI
Associate Dean, Practice and Community Engagement, University of Kentucky, Lexington, Kentucky

GUEST EDITORS

PATRICIA B. HOWARD, PhD, RN, CNAA, FAAN
Associate Dean for the MSN and Doctorate of Nursing Program, University of Kentucky College of Nursing, Lexington, Kentucky

PEGGY EL-MALLAKH, PhD, RN
Assistant Professor, University of Kentucky College of Nursing, Lexington, Kentucky

AUTHORS

ABIR K. BEKHET, PhD, RN, HSMI
Assistant Professor of Psychiatric and Mental Health Nursing, Marquette University College of Nursing, Milwaukee, Wisconsin

MARGARET H. BRACKLEY, PhD, RN, FAAN, FAANP
Professor, Department of Family and Community Health Systems, The University of Texas Health Science Center at San Antonio School of Nursing; Director, Center for Violence Prevention, San Antonio, Texas

KATHLEEN R. DELANEY, PhD, RN, PMH-NP
Professor of Nursing, Department of Community, Systems and Mental Health Nursing, Rush College of Nursing, Chicago, Illinois

PEGGY EL-MALLAKH, PhD, RN
Assistant Professor, University of Kentucky College of Nursing, Lexington, Kentucky

BRITTANY N. EVANS, BA, BSN, RN
Crisis Management Unit, Baptist East Hospital, Louisville, Kentucky

KATHERINE S. FABRIZIO, PhD
Physical Medicine and Rehabilitation, Birmingham Veterans Affairs Medical Center, Birmingham, Alabama

PATRICIA B. HOWARD, PhD, RN, CNAA, FAAN
Associate Dean for the MSN and Doctorate of Nursing Program, University of Kentucky College of Nursing, Lexington, Kentucky

STACEY M. INMAN, BSBA, JD, BSN, RN
University of Louisville School of Nursing, Louisville, Kentucky

NORMAN L. KELTNER, EdD, CRNP
Professor, School of Nursing, University of Alabama at Birmingham,
Birmingham, Alabama

KAREN M. ROBINSON, PhD, PMHCNS-BC, FAAN
Professor of Nursing, School of Nursing, University of Louisville, Louisville, Kentucky

JENNY L. SAULS, DSN, RN, CNE
Professor of Nursing, Associate Director for On-Ground Programs, School of Nursing,
Middle Tennessee State University, Murfreesboro, Tennessee

CELESTE SHAWLER, PhD, PMHCNS-BC
Associate Professor, School of Nursing, University of Louisville, Louisville, Kentucky

MARY LOU DELEON SIANTZ, PhD, RN, FAAN
Assistant Dean of Diversity and Cultural Affairs, University of Pennsylvania School of
Nursing, Philadelphia, Pennsylvania

M. JANE SURESKY, DNP, PMHCNS-BC
Assistant Professor of Psychiatric and Mental Health Nursing, Frances Payne Bolton
School of Nursing, Case Western Reserve University, Cleveland, Ohio

RUTH "TOPSY" STATEN, PhD, RN, PMH-CNS
Associate Professor, University of Kentucky, College of Nursing, Lexington, Kentucky

LITA F. WARISE, EdD, RN, CNE
Associate Professor of Nursing, School of Nursing, Middle Tennessee State University,
Murfreesboro, Tennessee

CHRISTINA C. WEI, PhD, RN
Postdoctoral Student in Family Psychiatric Mental Health Nurse Practitioner Program,
Department of Family and Community Health Systems, The University of Texas Health
Science Center at San Antonio School of Nursing, San Antonio, Texas

GAIL B. WILLIAMS, PhD, RN
Professor, Department of Family and Community Health Systems, The University of Texas
Health Science Center at San Antonio School of Nursing; Co-director, Center for Violence
Prevention, San Antonio, Texas

EDILMA L. YEARWOOD, PhD, RN, PMHCNS, BC, FAAN
Associate Professor, School of Nursing and Health Studies, Georgetown University,
Washington, DC

JACLENE A. ZAUSZNIEWSKI, PhD, RN-BC, FAAN
Kate Hanna Harvey Professor of Community Health Nursing and Associate Dean for
Doctoral Education, Frances Payne Bolton School of Nursing, Case Western Reserve
University, Cleveland, Ohio

Contents

This article describes what is known about mental health in children, adolescents, adults, and the elderly globally in high-, middle- and low-income countries. The social determinants of health are described as well as the paradigm shift from focusing on psychopathology to looking at ways in which individuals and communities can embrace mental health promotion to decrease stigma and provide care for all individuals in resource-rich and resource-poor environments. The need to expand the content in nursing curricula to include mental health concepts at all levels of training, foster mental health research, and promote international collaboration around best practices is also discussed.

If the health of children is to be improved, systems of care for youth must organize and collaborate around an emphasis toward promotion of health and prevention of mental illness. This approach demands an understanding of the complex interplay of genes, environment, risk, and protective factors that influence the manifestation of behavior problems. The focus of this article is prevention efforts aimed at processes thought to be involved in the development of mental illnesses. A particular emphasis is on prevention strategies that reduce risk prior to the onset of an identifiable mental disorder. Included are interventions appropriate to nurses who deal with children in schools, pediatric primary care, and specialty mental health care.

Chronic medical illness among children and adolescents is a growing concern with implications for informal and formal caregivers. When coupled with a psychiatric comorbidity, implications grow exponentially. Nurses who care for child and adolescent populations play a crucial role in optimizing physical and mental health when they interface with patients and their caregivers. Evidence-based interventions can promote positive outcomes and enhance quality of life, whereas failure to use evidence-based approaches has serious consequences to the health of youth with medical and psychiatric comorbidities.

Anxiety is a common feeling for patients and families during the critical care experience. As anxiety for critically ill patients presents increased risks for morbidity and mortality, it is imperative that nurses strive to identify unrelieved anxiety early to prevent adverse events. Alleviating anxiety experienced by families as a result of the critical care experience involves providing assurance, allowing them to remain near the patient, providing accurate and current information, providing for their comfort, and projecting a supportive attitude. As constant care providers, nurses can have the greatest impact on creating an environment that is safe, healing, and humane for critically ill patients and their families.

In greater numbers than in prior conflicts, service members deployed as part of Operation Enduring Freedom and Operation Iraqi Freedom have an increased risk of experiencing a traumatic brain injury (TBI). The basics of TBI are discussed, with particular attention paid to blast-related events, as this is a common mechanism of injury in this population. Particular attention is focused on the pharmacologic treatment of the sequlae of TBI and common comorbid conditions.

This article provides suggestions for skill development for substance abuse (SA) treatment agencies and providers for implementing Treatment Improvement Protocol number 25: Substance Abuse Treatment and Domestic Violence. Methods for detecting, screening, intervening, and referring victims and perpetrators of intimate partner violence enrolled in SA treatment are presented. Evidence-based brief intervention is presented. A 2-minute screen for domestic violence as well as danger assessment for lethality of abuse and the Conflict Tactics Scales 2 are reviewed. A survey of interventions aimed at establishing trust, brief intervention from best practice, guidelines for safety planning, compliance strategies for SA treatment, and community resource development are presented.

The physical health of people with schizophrenia is poor, and the challenges in finding effective treatment and optimizing health outcomes are significant. However, it is likely that people diagnosed with schizophrenia can be partners in the treatment of their physical health problems. Research suggests that many people with schizophrenia value physical health and will participate in health-related behaviors when they are provided with the opportunity to do so.

This integrative review summarizes current research on resilience in adult family members who have a relative with a diagnosed mental disorder that is considered serious. Within the context of resilience theory, studies identifying risk/vulnerability and positive/protective factors in family members are summarized, and studies examining seven indicators of resilience, including acceptance, hardiness, hope, mastery, self-efficacy, sense of coherence, and resourcefulness, are described. Implications for clinical practice and recommendations for future research are presented.

Americans are living longer than ever before in history. With age comes an increased risk for chronic mental health disorders. About 1 in 8 baby boomers is expected to be diagnosed with Alzheimer disease, which will amount to some ten million members of this age cohort. The prevalence of mental health disorders among the elderly is often unrecognized. One in four older adults lives with depression, anxiety disorders, or other significant psychiatric disorders. Mental health disorders are frequently comorbid in older adults, occurring with a number of common chronic illnesses such as in diabetes, cardiac disease, and arthritis. The public is becoming more aware of the aging of the population and the difficulties that are exacerbated by unmet services and limited access to mental health services. This article describes policy issues related to chronic mental health disorders and the older population. Mental health parity, a recent policy issue occurring at the national level, is discussed first followed by workforce issues specific to the discipline of nursing.

This article provides detailed information about assessing the mental health needs of older adults as well as strategies to maintain mental health. An overview of the public health needs of older adults is provided that includes examples of policies that ensure minimum physical and mental health for older adults. Multiple resources are described that will enable clinicians to access information that will increase their knowledge of assessment of mental health needs of older adults.

THE CLINICS ARE NOW AVAILABLE ONLINE!

Access your subscription at:
www.theclinics.com

Preface

Mental Health Across the Lifespan

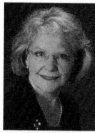 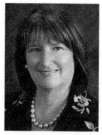

Patricia B. Howard, PhD, RN, CNAA, FAAN   Peggy El-Mallakh, PhD, RN
Guest Editors

A number of foundational principles have emerged in recent years to explain mental health and mental illness. Each is simply stated, yet each has profound importance for patients and nurses: 1) mental health is fundamental to overall health; 2) mental illnesses can occur at any age; and 3) the presence or absence of a mental illness has significant implications for functioning, well-being, and life satisfaction throughout a person's life.[1,2] Available statistics illuminate the prevalence of mental illnesses across the lifespan: almost 21% of children have a diagnosed mental illness, primarily anxiety, mood, or disruptive disorders. Similarly, the overall prevalence rate of mental illnesses among adults is about 21%, with the primary diagnoses being anxiety, particularly phobias and post-traumatic stress disorder, and major depressive disorder. Bipolar disorder and schizophrenia are less prevalent among adults, but have more serious consequences for overall functioning, well-being, and life satisfaction. Prevalence rates of mental illnesses among the elderly are about 19.8%, with anxiety disorders, severe cognitive disorders, and mood disorders as the most frequently diagnosed mental illnesses in this age group.[1]

A focus on a lifespan perspective in mental health necessarily leads to examination of a similar construct, that of the *life course*, which postulates that early life events influence future events.[3] In the case of mental illness, this suggests that untreated childhood mental illness and disadvantages—abuse, neglect, chronic illness, and emotional/behavioral problems with peers and in school—can set the stage for a lifetime of mental illness and maladaptive coping, including depression, post-traumatic stress disorder, and substance abuse. Indeed, researchers observe that in many cases, mental illness in adulthood first appeared prior to or during adolescence,[4] which underscores the importance of early recognition and treatment to optimize outcomes in future years.

Nurses are ideally positioned to recognize those at high risk for developing mental illnesses, promote mental health, and provide treatment for mental illnesses, not only

Nurs Clin N Am 45 (2010) ix–x
doi:10.1016/j.cnur.2010.08.001
0029-6465/10/$ – see front matter © 2010 Elsevier Inc. All rights reserved.

nursing.theclinics.com

at discrete time points in a patient's life—regardless of whether it occurs during childhood or advanced age—and over the trajectory of a person's life course. As guest editors, our goal for this issue of *Nursing Clinics of North America* is to provide direction for nurses to use the nursing process in all age groups and in a wide variety of contexts. The contributors have focused on a comprehensive review of mental health issues across the lifespan from a global perspective as well as contemporary, age-related issues that all health care providers encounter on a daily basis. For the child and adolescent populations, articles focus on comorbid medical and psychiatric illnesses and prevention of mental illnesses. For the adult population, the authors describe anxiety among patients treated in critical care units, traumatic brain injury in war veterans, medical illnesses in people with schizophrenia, resilience in family members of those with serious mental illnesses, and the interplay between substance abuse and intimate partner violence. Articles related to the elderly focus on social policy concerns and assessment and maintenance of mental health in this population.

Collectively, the articles illuminate the multiple and complex issues that all mental health care providers face in the treatment of mental illness. They also illustrate the importance of including psychiatric mental-health nursing content in curriculum at all levels and for all specialties because the lifespan treatment needs of this vulnerable population spans the health care system. Finally, we hope that the message that authors deliver prompts researchers and funding agencies to address gaps in our knowledge base about interventions so that nurses in direct care roles will have the information that they need to provide evidence-based treatment in their efforts to improve the quality of life for those who seek their care.

Patricia B. Howard, PhD, RN, CNAA, FAAN

Peggy El-Mallakh, PhD, RN

University of Kentucky College of Nursing
202 College of Nursing Building
760 Rose Street
Lexington, KY 40536-0232, USA

E-mail addresses:
pbhowa00@uky.edu (P. B. Howard)
peggy.el-mallakh@uky.edu (P. El-Mallakh)

REFERENCES

1. U.S. Department of Health and Human Services. Mental health: a report of the surgeon general—executive summary. Rockville, MD: U.S. Department of Health and Human Services, Substance Abuse and Mental Health Services Administration, Center for Mental Health Services, National Institutes of Health, National Institute of Mental Health, 1999.
2. Institute of Medicine. Improving the quality of health care for mental and substance-use conditions. Washington, DC: National Academies Press; 2006.
3. Berkman LF, Kawachi I. A historical framework for social epidemiology. In: Berkman LF, Kawachi I, editors. Social epidemiology. New York: Oxford University Press; 2000.
4. Jamieson KH, Romer D. A call to action. In: Evans DL, Foa EB, Gur RE, et al, editors. Treating and preventing adolescent mental health disorders: what we know and what we don't know. New York: Oxford University Press; 2005.

Global Issues in Mental Health Across the Life Span: Challenges and Nursing Opportunities

Edilma L. Yearwood, PhD, RN, PMHCNS, BC[a],*,
Mary Lou DeLeon Siantz, PhD, RN[b]

KEYWORDS

- Mental health nursing • Life span • Global burden of disease
- Social determinants of health • Paradigm shift • Primary care

SIGNIFICANCE

Mental health disorders significantly contribute to the global burden of disease (GBD), which quantifies the effect of mortality, morbidity, and disability for specific diseases. In 2001, noncommunicable neuropsychiatric disorders accounted for 12% of the GBD worldwide and that number is expected to increase significantly by 2020.[1] Among adults and the elderly, 5 of the 10 most frequently occurring disorders measured by disability-adjusted life years (DALYs) are unipolar depression, alcohol abuse, schizophrenia, bipolar disorder, and self-inflicted injuries.[2,3] Although the quality and accuracy of global aggregate data on the prevalence and treatment of behavioral and psychiatric disorders in adults and the elderly would be considered fair, what is known about behavioral and psychiatric disorders in children and adolescents globally is very limited. GBD epidemiologic studies have not been applied to this age group because of the lack of age appropriate data gathering tools, inconsistent data gathering capacity across nations, varying cultural beliefs about children and child mental health, and arguably a myopic priority on medical issues in children. Therefore, the psychiatric data on children and adolescents from low- and middle-income countries have been sparse, leaving us primarily with data from high-income countries that point

[a] School of Nursing & Health Studies, Georgetown University, 3700 Reservoir Road, NW, Washington, DC 20057-1107, USA
[b] University of Pennsylvania School of Nursing, Room 453 Fagin Hall, 418 Curie Boulevard, Philadelphia, PA 19104-4217, USA
* Corresponding author.
E-mail address: ely2@georgetown.edu

Nurs Clin N Am 45 (2010) 501–519
doi:10.1016/j.cnur.2010.06.004
0029-6465/10/$ – see front matter © 2010 Elsevier Inc. All rights reserved.

to a troubling picture of depression and high suicide rates, particularly in the adolescent population.[4,5]

About 25% of all persons will develop one or more psychiatric or behavioral disorders during their lifetime with depression the leading psychiatric disorder with respect to disability affecting all cultures, countries, and age groups across the life span.[6] This article provides an overview of what is currently known about mental health and mental illness across global communities and age groups, describes the global state of mental health nursing including challenges to growing the specialty of psychiatric-mental health nursing, and highlights recommendations for developing human resources to meet significant changes in mental health needs throughout the world.

URGENT NEED FOR A PARADIGM SHIFT

The World Health Organization (WHO) is credited with the statement, "There can be no health without mental health,"[7(p11)] a sentiment repeatedly endorsed by several international organizations who acknowledge the complex interplay of social, biologic, environmental, and economic factors that are the basis of mental health. The WHO and other concerned organizations and individuals have shifted their focus to identifying barriers to health equity, promoting mental health and prevention efforts, decreasing stigma, and identifying ways to empower individuals, families and communities. In many parts of the world, this is a significant shift from the traditional focus on the disease aspect of mental illness. Both psychiatric and generalist nurses in poorly resourced environments are in a unique position to play an active role in this shift from an illness model to one of individual, family and community education, empowerment, and prevention.

SOCIAL DETERMINANTS OF HEALTH: DRIVERS OF MENTAL HEALTH IN 2010 AND BEYOND

Social scientists, health care practitioners, researchers, and mental health proponents are increasingly advocating for large-scale social, political, and economic changes as a means to more effectively intervene to reduce health inequities that are impeding positive changes in health and mental health status and outcomes globally. The stark difference in resources available to leverage for health in high-income versus low- and middle-income countries is glaring and can no longer be ignored. Concerns about significant social justice issues and the need for health equity propelled the development of the *Social determinants of health* (SDH) document[8] and the philosophy of the WHO. The catalyst behind this paradigm shift is the need to address the known barriers to effective health and mental health care. Otherwise, there will be no significant change in the overall health of all global communities and populations.

Social determinants include economic status, living environments, gender equity, public policies, and local and national politics that either serve to maintain inequality or promote equity among its people. Population health, both medical and psychological, can be positively influenced in environments where there is economic growth, equitable distribution of power and resources, and equitable access to jobs. Furthermore, healthy living environments must be free of violence, overcrowded living and working spaces, pollutants, toxins, and diseases; must have a ready supply of clean water; and must provide accessible, affordable, health care services. The SDH advocates for principles outlined in **Box 1**.

For low- and middle-income countries, the SDH provides a framework for interventions at the individual, family, community, gender, policy, and national levels. At the

> **Box 1**
> **SDH principles target**
>
> 1. Improving conditions of daily life that effect birth, living environments, successful growth and development, work status, and health across all age groups
>
> 2. Equitable distribution of power, money and resources, which are the acknowledged structural drivers of access, hope, human and environmental resources, economic strength, and healthy societies
>
> 3. Education for all, a trained workforce, and public awareness about the social determinants of health; these 3 components must be present within population segments globally to empower the populous to effectively assess health problems, develop, demand, and implement action plans to support health and mental health, and to evaluate outcomes[8]

individual level, education must be available for all and healthy development of children must be supported through initiatives that enrich their social, emotional, physical, and psychological growth. At the family level, parent education should be available to support fragile individuals who may be overwhelmed with parenting responsibilities, lack knowledge about the needs of children, or who want to improve their parenting skills. At the community level, there must be thoughtful planning when creating communities to optimize spaces that are safe and which provide resources for exercise and recreation. There should also be areas to grow and manage food and secure and sustain a healthy water supply. Community planners must also be mindful of the relationship between adequate nutrition, learning, and overall health. They should strive to create and advocate for jobs that are accessible, within safe working environments, invoke low stress, and attainable by a variety of community members. Within this model, individuals who may be vulnerable because of age, gender, sexual orientation, religious affiliation, race, or mental illness would be protected by policies developed and enforced by the government. Policies would also ensure an adequate income level and would support basic human needs including health care. On the national level, governments would advocate for the health and mental health of their citizens by enacting incentives, policies, and programs that integrate the SDH principles and decrease the brain drain of educated health professionals fleeing to high-income and resource-rich countries.

MENTAL ILLNESS: EFFECT OF HEALTH INEQUITY ACROSS THE LIFE SPAN

Mental health is defined as a state of physical, emotional, social, and psychological well-being in which the individual is productive, able to adapt to changes or adversity, able to maintain fulfilling relationships with others, and contributes positively to society.[9,10] In contrast, mental illness refers to a diagnosable mental disorder that affects thinking, mood, behaviors, relationships with others, and ability to function.[9,11]

It is estimated that nearly 20% of all children globally have a disabling mental illness, with little attention paid to prevention and treatment of youngsters who experience disasters, wars, or undergo sexual, physical, and psychological abuse and abandonment.[3] With less than one-quarter of children believed to be receiving any type of psychiatric treatment,[12] it is no surprise that neuropsychiatric disorders continue into adulthood along with the development of serious comorbidities such as substance abuse, high-risk behaviors, obesity, anorexia, diabetes, and aggression.

Globally, untreated mental illness affects the individuals suffering from the disorder, family members, and the larger society. These parties may not only be burdened by the financial and caretaking toll involved but they may also lose the relational and productivity potential of the individual diagnosed with the disorder.

Although GBD neuropsychiatric disorders have considerable geographic variation in both occurrence and prognosis, they are found in every culture and country globally, are known for their early onset compared with other severe medical diseases, and have a course that is chronic in nature, thereby compromising the mental health of individuals across the life span.[13]

In general, global data about the magnitude of mental illness in children, adults, and the elderly are often offered as an estimate and therefore must be interpreted with caution because they are incomplete. Even so, the data are startling. The WHO[3] estimates that 450 million people worldwide experience one or more neuropsychiatric disorders. Between 66% and 90% of these individuals, who may never receive treatment, are primarily in low- and middle-income, resource-poor countries. They lack mental health treatment resources and access treatment later in the course of the disorder. This is a result of lack of knowledge, stigma, and reluctance to seek help from others. These individuals adhere poorly to treatment recommendations because of denial, poverty, or lack of access.[14]

Consistently the data show that the gap in treatment is in large part caused by stigma and lack of mental health treatment resources. The gap in accurate prevalence data is attributable to lack of adequate data gathering methods, variability in tools used to gather mental health data across countries, stigma toward the mentally ill resulting in low priority of mental health issues within and across countries, lack of resources, and uncertainty as to what to do with the data once this information is known.

Mental health resources receive roughly 1% of the health budget in low- and middle-income countries worldwide. As a result, those suffering from mental illnesses are not receiving current evidence-based treatment that has proven to be efficacious in high-income countries.[15] **Table 1** provides a list of the common mental health disorders and behaviors by age group, and the prognosis based on residence in low-, middle- or high-income countries.

Unipolar Depression

Cardiovascular disease and depression are the 2 leading causes of GBD worldwide. Depression is found in all age groups and across all cultures, however, variability in presentation may exist with depression. It is frequently comorbid with physical and chronic illnesses like cardiovascular disease as well as other psychiatric disorders. Risk factors for depression include poverty, family history, trauma, poor education, female gender, and multiple losses. Common symptoms include somatization, depressed mood, sleep and appetite disturbances, weight loss or weight gain, poor concentration, anhedonia, anertia, decreased libido, hopelessness, and thoughts of death.[16]

It is recommended that screening for depression in low- and middle-income countries and in high-income countries occur in primary health care settings and across all age groups because depressed individuals (1) rarely access psychiatric treatment early but may access medical care in the hope that a medical condition is causing their psychic discomfort; (2) are frequently in denial about the severity of their symptoms; and (3) are at risk for self-injury prompting the need for early case finding. Screening tools that are valid across cultures and in low- and middle-income countries include the General Health Questionnaire, the Kessler Distress Scale, and the Hopkins Symptom Checklist.[17]

Depression is one risk factor for suicide. The WHO compared global rates of suicide between 1950 and 2000 and found that the rate of suicide was higher in adults older than 45 years of age compared with those less than 45 years of age (60% to 40%) in

Table 1
Global burden of mental illness across the life span

Age	Common Disorders/ Behaviors	Treatment Prognosis in LMIC	Treatment Prognosis in HIC
Children (birth to 11 y)	Attachment disorder; autism; ADHD; anxiety; depression; PTSD; victims of violence; suicide	Poor	Fair to good
Adolescents (12–20 y)	Bipolar disorder; conduct disorder; substance abuse; unipolar depression; anxiety; victims and perpetrators of violence; PTSD; self mutilation; suicide	Poor	Fair to good
Adults (21–64 y)	Unipolar depression; substance abuse; bipolar disorder; schizophrenia; anxiety disorders; victims and perpetrators of abuse; PTSD	Poor	Fair to good
Elderly (65+ y)	Unipolar depression; Alzheimer dementia; anxiety disorders; victims of violence; suicide	Poor	Fair to good

Abbreviations: ADHD, attention deficit hyperactivity disorder; HIC, high-income countries; LMIC, low- and middle-income countries; PTSD, post traumatic stress disorder.

1950. In 2000, the rates were 45% in those 45 years of age and older compared with 55% in those aged 5 to 44 years.[18] Suicide has consistently been the third cause of death in adolescents[4] and the tenth cause of death overall. An estimated 800,000 to 1.2 million people globally commit suicide each year.[12,19]

In children and adolescents, depression may manifest through irritability, aggression, or poor school performance. In the elderly, depression may manifest as multiple and chronic complaints. Symptoms may be minimized or ignored by caretakers who focus on frailty, diabetes, coronary disease, or early dementia. Depression may be more pronounced in the elderly residing in nursing homes, those receiving home care services, and those living apart from children and other family members.[20]

Adolescents, adults, and the elderly may resort to self-medicating to manage depressive symptoms. Recommendations for those in low- and middle-income countries include early case finding through routine screening in primary care settings and during home visits by community workers, supportive psychoeducation groups conducted by trained community workers, use of generic antidepressants that are more affordable, and teaching problem-solving techniques and coping skills.[17]

Globally, research priorities for depressive disorders include evaluating effectiveness of cognitive-behavioral interventions across cultures, examining differences in effectiveness of interventions at the primary and secondary level of care, and assessing effectiveness of policies aimed at early detection and intervention.[21]

Alcohol and Other Drug Use and Dependence

GBD data on substance use highlight a notable trend that beginning at age 15 years, illicit drug use and alcohol contributes significantly to DALYs. Illicit substances include heroin, cocaine, cannabis, and amphetamines.[22] In the elderly, tobacco use accounted for higher mortality and DALYs than alcohol or illicit drugs.[23] However, alcohol is a factor in 36.4% of all psychiatric DALYs affecting those aged 15 to 29 years with males more significantly affected than females.[24]

The ICD-10 uses the criteria of hazardous, harmful, or dependence when describing the effects of alcohol use. Hazardous use poses physical, mental, social, or occupational risk for damage to the user or others. Harmful use is use that has already resulted in damage to health (ie, the individual has alcohol-induced pancreatitis) and dependent use is constant alcohol ingestion that effects behavior, physical health, cognition, relationships, and results in tolerance, withdrawal symptoms, and other harmful consequences.[25] Globally, the regions with the highest alcohol prevalence rates are the Americas, southeast Asia, and the Pacific region.[26]

Degenhardt and colleagues[22] conducted a large epidemiologic study on alcohol, cannabis, tobacco, and cocaine use on 54,069 participants from 17 countries. They found that higher income countries like the United States had the highest levels of use of all drugs and that strict antidrug policies did not deter use. In addition, results indicate that mid to late adolescence is a risk factor for initiation of substance use. Although females use substances less than males, there is a noticeable increase in the rate of use among females.

Substance dependence treatment recommendations in low- and middle-income countries include early screening (with tools such as the AUDIT, which has demonstrated reliability and validity across cultures) in primary care and brief intervention with follow-up and supportive services incorporated in community models of care. For success in low- and middle-income countries, additional and focused training of health care providers and community support workers would need to occur. In high-income countries, cognitive-behavioral therapy, 12-step approaches, pharmacotherapy, and motivation therapies were effective treatment strategies to use with alcoholics.[26] The priorities for research in this population include evaluating the effectiveness of strategies to decrease consumption in high-risk groups, evaluating the effectiveness of early detection and brief intervention models, and evaluating long-term efficacy of treatment delivered across different treatment settings.[21]

Schizophrenia

Worldwide, the incidence of schizophrenia is 1.5 per 10,000 individuals.[27,28] It is estimated that there are nearly 42 million people in low- and middle-income countries who meet the ICD-10 and DSM-IV criteria for schizophrenia.[27] These criteria include odd-eccentric behaviors, thought disorder (delusions, illusions), misperceptions (hallucinations), negative symptoms such as avolition, blunted affect, apathy, social withdrawal, and incoherent speech.[16,27] Individuals with schizophrenia have high mortality and morbidity compared with other neuropsychiatric disorders because of increased risk for suicide, higher prevalence of diabetes and cardiovascular disease secondary to metabolic syndrome, higher rates of smoking, comorbid substance use, obesity and adverse reactions to psychotropic medications.[27]

Within the SDH model of care, the recommended intervention at the individual and family level focuses on individuals with schizophrenia and their family members. Interventions include early case finding, treatment in the community, brief hospitalization when needed to stabilize acute symptoms, teaching about symptoms of relapse and the importance of medication adherence, and patient and family education about the illness. At the community level, education and social marketing campaigns focus on reducing stigma surrounding the disorder and on developing and enforcing supportive policies.[29] The Lancet Global Mental Health Group advocates for research on (1) effectiveness and safety of community health care workers dispensing antipsychotic medications, (2) effectiveness of culturally informed rehabilitation services and community-based treatment programs in reducing stigma, and (3) changes in access to care for individuals with psychotic disorders.[21]

Dementia

Alzheimer disease (AD) is the most common cause of dementia. AD effects approximately 5 million people annually[30] and results in institutionalization, caregiver role strain, and diminished quality of life. Developing countries bear the highest burden of older individuals with dementia with almost 3 times the number compared with developed countries.[30,31] Data from high-income countries recommend early diagnosis, instituting interventions to maintain physical health and activity, treating behavioral and psychological symptoms, and providing respite and support for family caregivers.[7] Recommendations for dementia care in low- and middle-income countries include (1) integration with comorbid chronic disease care in primary care, (2) development of advocacy efforts and use of scarce resources to develop community programs to support individuals with AD, (3) training of community health care workers in early screening using valid tools such as the Mini-mental State Examination, and (4) provisions for education, support, and management strategies for family members along with community health care workers.

A survey of 500 individuals with AD and their 614 caretakers was conducted in 6 countries to obtain information on quality of life and information gaps for those dealing with the disease.[32] Participants indicated that the most important factors for them included maintaining the best possible quality of life, safety, receiving treatment to control symptoms, learning about easy to implement management regimens, and timely receipt of information about AD.

Violence

Globally, significant differences in rates of violence exist based on gender, age, culture, and income. Violence, a major public health concern, includes intimate partner violence, suicide, self-inflicted injuries without mortality, homicide, child abuse and neglect, elder abuse, war, sexual abuse, and community violence perpetrated frequently by youth. Statistics from the *World health report on violence and health*[33] indicated that 1.6 million lives were lost to violence, with another 16 million injuries resulting from violent acts in 2000. The report also stated that low- and middle-income countries have more than twice the GBD consequences associated with violence than high-income countries. The ecological model identifies 5 factors used to understand the phenomena of violence: individual biologic, relational, sociocultural, community environments, and the larger societal context.[33]

Violence against women and children

Women and children are among the most vulnerable victims of societal violence. The incidence of violence toward these 2 groups is significant and includes sexual violence, physical violence, psychological violence, genital mutilation, war crimes of rape, forced family separation, migration, and trafficking. Stigma, cultural beliefs about the role and value of women and children, power imbalances, and lack of human and health care resources contribute to the paucity of attention paid to the long-term consequences of violence and trauma in these victims. Consequences include the effects on overall mental health, self-concept, changes in behavioral and psychological symptoms, poorer quality of life, and changes in relationships and relatedness to others. Recommendations for intervening in gender-based violence include conducting multidisciplinary and culture-specific research and public awareness campaigns, empowering women economically and through education, and developing and adhering to international policies that hold perpetrators of gender-based violence accountable for their actions.[34] Other violence prevention recommendations include ownership of violence prevention at the national and community levels, increasing data collection on prevalence and research on the cultural context of violence, comprehensive advocacy for all victims, and a strong and consistent global response to violence within a human rights context.[33]

Suicide

Suicide as an act of violence against the self claims the lives of approximately 1 million individuals worldwide annually with a mortality rate of 16 per 100,000. For every successful suicide, there are multiple survivors of attempts. Risk factors for suicide include depression, schizophrenia, substance abuse, age, and male gender. Suicide is the tenth cause of death globally, the second cause of death in those aged 10 to 24 years, the third cause of death in those aged 15 to 44 years, is more prevalent in China, Belarus, Lithuania, and Cuba, and on the increase in both men and women older than 75 years of age.[3,4,18] Recommendations for intervening to reduce the suicide rates include launching public awareness campaigns about the scope of the problem and warning signs, reducing access to common highly lethal methods such as firearms and toxic pesticides, and training primary health care providers to screen for suicide ideation, intent, and risk. In addition, it is recommended that interventions to treat and strengthen support networks for survivors of suicide attempts begin early.

DISORDERS SPECIFIC TO CHILDREN AND ADOLESCENTS

As stated previously, global epidemiologic data on child and adolescent behavioral and psychiatric disorders are inconsistent and are frequently presented as an estimate of the problem because of cultural barriers, an absence of a national focus on the mental health needs of this age group, and poor data gathering tools specific to this population. In 2005, the WHO used a survey instrument to gather information about youth services, provider resources, and training of workers involved in child mental health. Key informants in 192 countries were sent the instrument; 66 responded for a response rate of approximately 33%. Surveys were not sent to informants in the United States, France, Australia, or Canada, as these are viewed as high-income countries with well-established resources. Although there were inconsistencies and missing data in some of the surveys returned, the Atlas was seen as an initial attempt to collect data in several crucial areas. Despite the study limitations, results from the data collected highlighted the gaps in services for this population. Specific findings indicated (1) there was a paucity of trained health care providers; (2) information about childhood disorders was lacking; and (3) planned programs, treatment services, and policies that advocate for children were essentially nonexistent. Missing too were country-specific data with sufficient financial support in low- and middle-income countries to yield positive outcomes.[4,12]

Approximately 20% of children and adolescents are believed to have a diagnosable psychiatric disorder; 50% of adults report that their mental illness originated in childhood.[4] Childhood psychiatric disorders are frequently described in terms of internalizing (depression, anxiety, autism, psychosis,) versus externalizing (attention deficit hyperactivity, conduct disorder, aggression, oppositional) behaviors. Risk factors for child and adolescent behavioral and mental illness include poverty, poor attachment, physical and sexual abuse and neglect, family history of mental illness, genetics, substance abuse, child soldiering, residing in war-torn and violent environments, displacement, and the direct and indirect effects of human immunodeficiency virus (HIV) and AIDS.[4,5]

WHO RECOMMENDATIONS TO ADDRESS MENTAL HEALTH TREATMENT GAPS

The WHO has been at the forefront internationally in highlighting the significant disparities that exist between medical and neuropsychiatric disorders. In an effort to address disparities, the WHO has made recommendations concerning mental health based on their assessment of both high-income countries and low- and middle-income countries. Recommendations are concerned with assessment, treatment, sites of care, education and training, as well as policy and research (**Box 2**).

Compliance with these recommendations would offer a unique and fruitful opportunity to develop and promote the practice, education, and research base of all psychiatric and mental health professionals, especially nurses. In addition, nurses would have more opportunities to provide services to individuals, groups, and communities throughout the life span using a community participatory and health promotion framework. Mental health promotion must become a valued part of the global development language, a priority in our public health discourse, research agendas, and a foundation for primary care.

GLOBAL MENTAL HEALTH NURSING: CURRENT TRENDS

Mental health nursing, an essential component of health care in general, has often been overlooked among low- and middle-income countries with inadequate

---

Box 2
Addressing treatment gaps

1. Mental health assessment and treatment should be accessible in primary care
2. Psychotropic medications need to be readily available, accessible and affordable to all who would benefit from them
3. Mental health care needs to move from institutional settings into communities
4. Public education about mental illness and mental health needs to occur
5. Families, communities, and consumers should be involved in advocacy, policy-making, and in the development of self-help groups
6. National mental health programs need to be established and financially supported
7. The training of mental health care professionals should be increased and improved
8. Links with other governmental and nongovernmental institutions should be increased
9. Mental health systems should be monitored using quality indicators
10. Additional support needs to be in place for mental health research[3]

recruitment, insufficient training, and a lack of emphasis on the unique and crucial skills of this nursing specialty. Consequently, worldwide, the number of mental health nurses available to meet the overwhelming demand for skilled mental health treatment and mental health promotion is low. Low-income countries have the smallest number of mental health nurses and they tend to work primarily in older traditional mental health hospitals with limited human and material resources.[35] The preparation and continuing education of mental health nurses in these countries frequently fails to include new knowledge and skills needed to meet the complex and evolving mental health needs of the population. Therefore, the importance of global mental health nursing has never been greater than it is currently.

Nurses not only play a critical role in providing timely, effective, and comprehensive services but more importantly, they promote and advocate for mental health, and prevention of behavioral and mental health disorders.[10] Nurses in developing countries increasingly provide mental health care to those in need in isolated settings and with limited education. They experience limited support through national policies or from other mental health professionals. On the other hand, mental health nurses in high-income countries play a critical role in planning, developing, and delivering mental health care at various sites including primary health care, hospitals, community clinics, and schools. In developed countries, nurses are the main providers in the health care system and are a critical resource in countries planning to improve their mental health services.[35]

MENTAL HEALTH NURSING CHALLENGES

Major challenges to global mental health nursing are attributed to lack of interest in the field, lack of incentives to pursue a mental health nursing career, and stigma and taboos associated with this fragile and vulnerable population. Stigma surrounding mental illness and the perceived low status of psychiatric nursing continues to be a problem in recruitment and retention of nurses into this specialty.[35] Retention of nurses in general and psychiatric nurses in particular has been problematic in low- and middle-income countries. The reasons cited include nurse migration to other countries, nurses choosing to leave the profession entirely, a lack of safety and security in the work environment, and the general shortage of adequately trained nurses and support staff. Workplace violence has also had a significant effect on recruitment and retention worldwide, ultimately affecting student decisions not to become mental health nurses.[36]

GLOBAL MENTAL HEALTH NURSING ENVIRONMENTS
Primary Care

As a strategy to close the treatment gap and provide needed mental health services, integrating mental health into primary care has been recommended by the WHO.[8,37] The use of this already existing resource is seen as an affordable investment that must be supported by service coordination, development and integration of services, and use of community-specific practice models.

Nurses are the primary service providers in many countries, providing most of the health care in resource-strapped countries. In many countries where there are few psychiatrists, nurses actively provide mental health services in primary care; however, additional education and resources must be allocated for these nurses to develop mental health assessment and treatment skills. Nigeria is an example of this type of environment where nurses provide a range of services that include consultation, counseling, psychotherapy, home visits, referrals, and follow-up after treatment. Nurses evaluate the patient's environment and serve as care coordinators across multiple systems. They also encourage and facilitate active participation by family caretakers in the treatment process because the family caretaker is frequently the only available resource to manage the day-to-day needs of the mentally ill individual.[38]

Although several countries, especially in Europe, use a general health care model of integrating mental health into primary care, there is a continuing need to increase the availability of mental health care in communities and to strengthen the level of integration of mental health care in primary care.[12,35] The move to treat mental illness in communities is propelled by several issues including human rights abuse experienced within many treatment institutions, psychological deterioration of individuals maintained long-term in institutions, and the exacerbation of stigma that accompanies a stay in psychiatric facilities.[12] Panama with a population of nearly 3 million, one-third of whom live in poverty, faced multiple challenges in the integration of mental health into primary care. Mental health nurses in this country established local, national, and international partnerships to assess mental health needs, identified quality practice indicators, and established an action agenda to improve mental health practice and service delivery in mental health and primary care settings.[39]

Psychiatric Hospitals

Traditionally, nurses have been critical members of teams that provide care for persons with mental disorders through direct care and case management. Although nurses make up the largest numbers in mental health interdisciplinary teams in psychiatric hospitals, they work alongside other mental health professionals including psychiatrists, psychologists, social workers, activity therapists, and psychiatric technicians.

Noteworthy changes have occurred in recent decades in the care and management of mentally ill individuals including deinstitutionalization of patients into the community, resulting in the closure of many psychiatric hospitals.[40] This practice is not universal and has been problematic. Lack of adequate community treatment resources and support for patients, poor planning for adequate preparation of patients in life skills, and failure to properly educate the community to these changes have impeded the success of these efforts. Some countries that have maintained their psychiatric hospitals have started to focus on changes within that environment to promote skill building in patients, improve institutional safety for patients and staff, and offer more humane treatment.[41]

For example, Norway has moved to an integrated mental health care model that was driven by closing of psychiatric hospitals, reduction of inpatient beds, deinstitutionalization, responsiveness to patient rights advocates, and a national mental health program endorsed by policy makers that advocated for community-based services.[42] However, many of the psychiatric hospitals in developing countries are not centrally located, not easily accessible, and are often accessed as a last resort. Unfortunately, some hospitals still operate under legislation that is more penal than therapeutic and places barriers to admission and timely discharge.[3] Regardless of the treatment setting, the ideal nursing role includes mental health assessment of needs, planning, implementation and evaluation of evidenced-based therapeutic interventions to promote optimal behavioral and psychological change, and active collaboration with the interdisciplinary mental health team, the patient, and the family.[41]

Community Mental Health

Community mental health interventions occur in a wide array of settings and at different levels of care. Services provided by nurses and other mental health professionals including paraprofessionals, should ideally link general inpatient mental health services with primary care services and informal care providers working in the community. Services can include rehabilitation, medication management, knowledge and skill development, crisis intervention and stabilization, and direct treatment. These interventions, which should be culturally adapted, can occur in therapeutic and supervised residential settings, home health, schools, employment settings, and other nontraditional sites.[43]

An exemplary model that received the 2008 MacArthur Foundation Award for Creative and Effective Community Interventions is the MANAS program in India, which serves as a vehicle to integrate care of common mental and behavioral disorders into primary care. With the use of external expert practitioners, a resource manual was developed to assist community health counselors in learning the essential skills needed to deliver mental health services for common disorders within their community. The manual contains nontechnical information in a structured and guided format on recognizing, assessing, and intervening in the management of depression and anxiety.[44]

Despite the shortage of nurses, community mental health nursing in some countries is having a positive effect. Advocates for these changes have included the WHO and the Pan American Health Organization (PAHO), which have mobilized a cadre of nurses in strategic positions in several countries. In low- and middle-income countries, a need was identified to change patient models of care from a biologic medical model (illness and disease focus) to a person-centered preventative approach with expansion of services to specific vulnerable groups. In the community these groups include children, adolescents, the elderly, forensics, and persons with comorbid conditions. This new model calls for greater patient, family, and caretaker involvement in learning about their illness and participation in illness management decisions. Keeping the individual who is experiencing psychiatric symptoms in the community and closer to family, friends, and community supports is a core element of this model. Recommended services include mental health promotion, education, and advocacy that decreases the stigma associated with mental illness while increasing awareness of mental health needs and care in the community. This approach takes behavioral and psychiatric disorders from the hidden halls of institutions to open arenas within the community.[1,35,45] These goals are consistent with the Psychiatric-Mental Health Nursing Scope and Standards of Practice as written and endorsed by the American Nurses Association (ANA), the American Psychiatric Nurses Association (APNA), and the International Society of Psychiatric-Mental Health Nurses (ISPN).[46]

GLOBAL MENTAL HEALTH NURSING IN THE FUTURE
New Paradigms

Four hundred and fifty million persons suffer from mental and behavioral disorders worldwide, and psychiatric disorders are projected to account for more than 15% of the total GBD by 2020. The only sustainable means of reducing the burden caused by such disorders will be prevention and mental health promotion.[1] Mental health nurse scientists will be needed to build the evidence that promotes best practices in complex and low-resource global communities; to integrate results gathered through worldwide collaborative partnerships with other nurse scientists, educators, practitioners, community members, and policy makers; and to evaluate and publish outcome data in both professional and lay journals and other popular print materials.

Evidenced-based Prevention

Preventive mental health has been in place for more than a century, beginning with the mental hygiene movement at the start of the twentieth century, which focused on prevention of behavioral problems and mental disorders in children and adults. These early strategies were transformed into experimental activities in primary health care, schools, and public health practices. However, the systematic development of a science-based prevention program with controlled studies to test for efficacy and feasibility did not begin until the 1980s.[47]

Most recently, research has focused on malleable risk and protective factors that reduce the incidence and prevalence of some mental health disorders as well as nursing interventions that promote mental health. Preventive interventions are deemed successful if they reduce risk factors and enhance protective factors associated with poor mental health. Prevention, a broad and complex concept, aims to reduce the incidence, prevalence, recurrence or quantity of time that the individual experiences symptoms, to decrease the risk factors that may trigger a mental illness, and minimize the effects of the illness on the affected person, their family, and society.[1,48]

The distinction between prevention and promotion is in the targeted outcome. Mental health disorder prevention targets the reduction of symptoms. It uses mental health promotion strategies as a means to achieve this goal. Mental health promotion aims to enhance positive mental health in the community with a secondary outcome of decreasing the incidence of mental disorders. Positive mental health is a powerful protective factor that protects against mental illness. These concepts overlap and are interrelated components of overall mental health.[49]

Evidenced-based Mental Health Promotion

Mental health itself is a resource for mental health promotion and is a basic human right that is essential for social and economic welfare. The overall goal is to transform the social determinants of health to increase affirming conditions that support mental health, reduce inequities, build social capital, effect positive changes in health, and narrow the gap in health expectancy between countries and within groups.[50] Interventions that promote mental health support everyone: those not currently at risk, those at increased risk, and those suffering or recovering from mental health alterations.[45] Mental health promotion activities imply the design of individual, social, and environmental conditions that enable optimal psychological and psychophysiologic development. Interventions should support the process of empowering others to achieve mental health, enhance their quality of life, increase capacity, and narrow the gap in health expectancy between countries and groups. It is an enabling process in collaboration with the entire community.[51] Mental health intervention research is needed on culturally sensitive topics, reducing stigma, community-based care strategies for individuals across the life span, quality of outcomes based on use of different types of care providers, and efficacy of different models of care in a variety of settings.[41,45]

Evidence-based Mental Health Policies

The WHO[43] has developed guidelines for mental health policy development. It is based on evidence that integrates values, principles, and assumptions about mental health. Such policies must be built on the mental health needs of populations and evidence-based mental health interventions that are integrated into a plan based on the country-specific vision for the mental health of its citizenry. To date, robust mental health policies are absent in more than 25% of countries, affecting nearly 31% of the global population. Usher and Grigg[41] identified that in some countries, mental health legislation was passed before 1960, rendering it outdated. Since 1990, an additional 51% of countries have passed varying levels of mental health legislation, which should be reviewed periodically for ongoing relevance and applicability.

Public policies that support prevention and health promotion based on community- and group-specific evidence are needed. With appropriate education, training, and collaborative research relationships with international partners, mental health nurses in low- and middle-income countries can have a significant effect on research, policy, and interventions to promote mental health within their own communities. With the stressor of poverty contributing to lack of resources, the development of mental disorders and limited employment opportunities, economic policies that promote economic prosperity are more likely to have a positive effect on the mental health of communities and, in turn, on individuals.[52] The need has never been greater for the development of comprehensive community mental health services and the integration of mental health into primary care using a broad public health framework that reflects the complex interrelationship between physical and mental health.

In New Zealand, the National Framework for Mental Health Nursing was created to sustain a mental health nursing workforce that promotes recovery and best practices. The framework, developed in 2005, provides strategic direction for the future of mental health nursing. The intent is to strengthen both nursing leadership and practice within a multidisciplinary clinical environment. The New Zealand Ministry of Health facilitated the establishment of the framework with advice from an expert mental health panel. The framework focuses on nursing leadership, the development and widespread use of practitioners, development and use of standards of care and practice, clinical career pathway opportunities, support for nursing education and research, and the recruitment and retention of nurses.[53]

Leading Mental Health Policy Development

Nursing leadership is needed more than ever in all countries to inspire innovation and risk taking to develop legislation that will transform mental health treatment, mental health nursing, and mental health policies. The challenge in addressing policy gaps is within reach if nurses who are aware of treatment and community needs are willing to become engaged in leading changes in capacity building, education, research, advocacy, and organizational infrastructures.[45,54] Risk and creativity require initiatives beyond the comfort zone of familiar solutions and traditions. Mental health nurses will need to begin by becoming more committed to understanding the mental health infrastructure and public policies within their own countries, collaborating to build the evidence needed to formulate policies, and disseminating the evidence collected from innovative and effective mental health research and interventions that are based on community participation. Nurses need to identify and communicate with key government officials who influence mental health, collaborate with key consumer advocacy groups, and partner with interdisciplinary organizations to advocate for strong mental health policies. To promote this level of mental health policy transformation, leadership skills will need to become a core component of mental health nursing education. In the United States, the practice doctorate (DNP) was developed to prepare nurses with advanced competencies for dealing with complex clinical, organizational, systems, and leadership roles. These nurses are expected to engage in clinical research to improve health care patient outcomes, design innovative and consumer-preferred programs, and develop, implement, and evaluate health policy at different levels of the health care system.[55] Unfortunately, nursing development in some countries has been hampered by lack of role models, limited definition of scope of practice, and poor reimbursement structures that do not serve as incentives to remain in the profession in the country where there is the greatest need for nurses or to pursue higher education and professional development.[56]

Mental Health Nursing Education

The recognition that care of persons with mental illness is complex and can be best delivered within a community or home setting has led to a need to change nursing curricula to include more theory and practice hours in mental health. For example, in Nigeria, a recommendation was proposed to provide mental health specialization after basic education so that nurse specialists could provide more "relevant and cost effective care."[38] In some countries, preparation for psychiatric nursing practice occurs after basic or graduate level; in others, targeted mental health programs are found at the preservice level, and in a third model, mental health concepts are woven throughout other core courses.[57] The profession, practice standards, and quality of care would benefit from a model of consistency in basic training in psychiatric-mental health nursing.

Mental health must be a core component of basic nursing education globally along with strong efforts to develop and support advanced practice degrees in mental health nursing. With a global shortage of psychiatrists and child psychiatrists, advanced practice nurses providing services in low- and middle-income countries would be invaluable in meeting the mental health needs of the population. Countries that do have advanced practice mental health nurses have shown that this type of health care practitioner can help contain cost, improve care, provide services to the most vulnerable, decrease the wait time to access services, and promote overall health.[56] Because no standard for mental health nursing education currently exists in most countries, curricula vary considerably. Standardization of basic curricula should be attempted and should include assessment of mental disorders, treatment, principles of rehabilitation, prevention, and mental health promotion. Ethical, legal, and research issues are more frequently included in the nursing curricula of high-income countries, but we would argue that, at the very least, aspects of these topics are critical concepts that all mental health nurses working in low- and middle-income countries should know.

Development of human resources in mental health is among the top 10 recommended actions for global mental health according to the *World health report of 2001*.[3] Recommended action steps range from relatively low-resource development (psychiatrists and psychiatric nurses) to mid-level development (educational centers for the preparation of a pool of mental health professionals), and high-level development (ongoing evidence-based advanced treatment skill development).

Educating the global nursing community about mental health requires administrative support and a critical mass of faculty who are committed to curriculum transformation throughout the planning and implementation process.

SUMMARY

Accurate global data about the extent of psychiatric and behavioral disorders in children and adults across the life span is lacking. Issues of stigma, poor and inconsistent data collection methodology, and socioeconomic variability affecting human and material resources all contribute to the gaps that exist in available prevalence data, access to treatment, and effectiveness of interventions within and across nations in those experiencing changes in their mental health status. What is clear is that the picture of mental health is vastly different in high-income countries compared with low- and middle-income countries for adults and children. In response to these glaring health inequities, the WHO, mental health advocates, and resource-poor communities have begun to focus on a new paradigm that moves away from a traditional pathologic view of mental illness. Instead, they strive to decrease the stigma surrounding mental illness and empower individuals in communities to develop community programs to intervene in managing psychiatric and behavioral needs while holding local and national governments accountable for the development and enforcement of policies to equitably support both the health and mental health needs of its citizenry.

Nurses globally have an opportunity to significantly affect the care and treatment of individuals across the life span who are in need of support to achieve mental health. Nurses have long been the profession that has led the way in working with communities to provide crucial public health care. In accepting the view that there is no health without mental health, the nursing profession globally can and should focus on developing the skills needed by all nurses and student nurses to provide both physical and mental health care to all individuals. Nursing, the largest health care profession, is in a unique position to aggressively intervene to address global health disparities that exist in the specialty of mental health.

ACKNOWLEDGMENTS

The authors wish to thank Dr Silvina Malvarez, Pan American Health Organization (PAHO) Regional Advisor for Nursing for her help in the development and refinement of this manuscript.

REFERENCES

1. World Health Organization. Prevention of mental disorders, effective interventions and policy options. Geneva (Switzerland): WHO; 2004.
2. Mathers C, Loncar D. Projections of global mortality and burden of disease from 2002 to 2030. PLoS Med 2006;3(11):e442.
3. World Health Organization. The world health report 2001, mental health: new understanding, new hope. Geneva (Switzerland): WHO; 2001.
4. Belfer M. Child and adolescent mental disorders: the magnitude of the problem across the globe. J Child Psychol Psychiatry 2008;49(3):226–36.
5. Patel V, Flisher A, Hetrick S, et al. Mental health of young people: a global public-health challenge. Lancet 2007;369(9569):1302–13.
6. Kastrup M, Ramos A. Global mental health. Dan Med Bull 2007;1(54):42–3.
7. World Health Organization. Mental health: facing the challenges, building solutions. Report from the WHO European Ministerial Conference. Copenhagen (Denmark): World Health Organization; 2005.
8. World Health Organization. Closing the gap in a generation. Health equity through action on the social determinants of health. Geneva (Switzerland): World Health Organization; 2008.
9. US Department of Health and Human Services. Mental health: a report of the surgeon general. Rockville (MD): US Department of Health and Human Services; 1999.
10. World Health Organization. Mental health: strengthening mental health promotion. 2007. Available at: http://www.who.int/mediacentre/factsheets/fs220/en/print.html. Accessed December 5, 2009.
11. National Alliance on Mental Illness. What is mental illness: mental illness facts. 2009. Available at: http://www.nami.org/. Accessed December 5, 2009.
12. World Health Organization. Atlas child and adolescent mental health resources, global concerns: implications for the future. Geneva (Switzerland): World Health Organization; 2005.
13. Andlin-Sobocki P, Jonsson B, Wittchen HU, et al. Cost of disorders of the brain in Europe. Eur J Neurol 2005;12(Suppl 1):1–27.

14. Kohn R, Saxena S, Levav I, et al. The treatment gap in mental health care. Bull World Health Organ 2004;82(11):858–66.
15. Patel V. Mental health in low- and middle-income countries. Br Med Bull 2007;81 & 82:81–96.
16. American Psychiatric Association. Diagnostic and statistical manual of mental disorders. 4th edition. Washington, DC: American Psychiatric Association; 2000.
17. Patel V, Simon G, Chowdhary N, et al. Packages of care for depression in low and middle-income countries. PLoS Med 2009;6(10):e1000159.
18. WHO. Suicide prevention (SUPRE). 2009. Available at: http://www.who.int/mental_health/prevention/suicide/suicideprevent/en/print.html. Accessed October 9, 2009.
19. Prince M, Patel V, Saxena S, et al. No health without mental health. Lancet 2007; 370(9590):859–77.
20. Chapman DP, Perry GS. Depression as a major component of public health for older adults. Prev Chronic Dis 2008;5(1). Available at: http://www.cdc.gov/pcd/issues/2008/jan/07_0150.htm. Accessed June 23, 2010.
21. Lancet Global Mental Health Group. Scale up services for mental disorders: a call for action. Lancet 2007;370(9594):1241–52.
22. Degenhardt L, Whiteford H, Hall W, et al. Estimating the burden of disease attributable to illicit drug use and mental disorders: what is "global burden of disease 2005" and why does it matter? Addiction 2009;104:1466–71.
23. Rehm J, Taylor B, Room R. Global burden of disease from alcohol, illicit drugs and tobacco. Drug Alcohol Rev 2006;25:503–13.
24. Rehm J, Mathers C, Popova S, et al. Global burden of disease and injury and economic cost attributable to alcohol use and alcohol-use disorders. 2009. Available at: www.thelancet.com. Accessed June 23, 2010.
25. World Health Organization. The ICD-10 classification of mental and behavioral disorders. Geneva (Switzerland): World Health Organization; 1992.
26. Benegal V, Chand P, Obot I. Packages of care for alcohol use disorder in low and middle-income countries. PLoS Med 2009;6(10):e1000170.
27. Mari J, Razzouk D, Thara R, et al. Packages of care for schizophrenia in low- and middle-income countries. PLoS Med 2009;6(10):e1000165.
28. Saha S, Chant D, Welham J, et al. A systematic review of the prevalence of schizophrenia. 10.137/journal.pmed.0020141. PLoS Med 2005;2(5):e141.
29. Rossler W, Salize HJ, Os J, et al. Size of burden of schizophrenia and psychotic disorders. Eur Neuropsychopharmacol 2005;15:399–409.
30. Ferri C, Prince M, Brayne C, et al. Global prevalence of dementia: a Delphi consensus study. Lancet 2005;366:2112–7.
31. Mathew R, Mathuranath RM. Issues in evaluation of cognition in the elderly in developing countries. Ann Indian Acad Neurol 2008;11:82–8.
32. Kurz A, Schulz M, Reed P, et al. Personal perspectives of persons with Alzheimer's disease and their carers: a global survey. Alzheimers Dement 2008;4: 345–52.
33. World Health Organization. World health report on violence and health. Geneva (Switzerland): WHO; 2002.
34. Russo N, Pirlott A. Gender-based violence concepts, methods and findings. Ann N Y Acad Sci 2006;1087:178–205.
35. World Health Organization. Atlas: nurses in mental health 2007. Geneva (Switzerland): World Health Organization; 2007.
36. Happell B, Cowin L, Roper C, et al. Introducing mental health nursing. A consumer-oriented approach. Crows Nest (Australia): Allen & Unwin; 2008.

37. World Health Organization. Integrating mental health into primary care, a global perspective. Geneva (Switzerland): World Health Organization; 2008.

38. World Health Organization. Ugochukwu C. Quality improvement of mental health, in Panama. In: Atlas: nurses in mental health. Geneva (Switzerland): World Health Organization; 2007. p. 44.

39. Raphel S, Yearwood E. Quality improvement of mental health care in Panama. In: World Health Organization. Atlas: nurses in mental health. Geneva (Switzerland): World Health Organization; 2007. p. 16.

40. Ash D, Benson A, Dunbar L, et al. Mental health services in Australia. In: Meadows G, Singh B, Grigg M, editors. Mental health in Australia: collaborative community practice. 2nd edition. Melbourne (Australia): Oxford University Press; 2007. p. 63–98.

41. Usher K, Grigg M. Mental health nursing trends and issues. Geneva (Switzerland): International Council of Nurses; 2009.

42. Pedersen B, Kolstad A. De-institutionalization and trans-institutionalization-changing trends of inpatient care in Norwegian mental health institutions 1950-2007. Int J Ment Health Syst 2009;3(28). DOI: 10.1186/1752-4458-3-28.

43. World Health Organization. Organization of services for mental health, mental health and service guidance package. Geneva: WHO; 2003. p. 14–6.

44. Sangath (n.d.). Manual for health counselors. Available at: www.sangath.com/sangath/files/otherpdfs/MANAS-health-counselor-training-manual-draft.pdf. Accessed November 10, 2009.

45. World Health Organization. Promoting mental health, concepts, emerging evidence and practice. Geneva (Switzerland): World Health Organization; 2004.

46. American Nurses Association. Psychiatric-mental health nursing: scope and standards of practice. Silver Springs (MD): American Nurses Association; 2007.

47. Hosman C, Llopis E, Saxena S. Prevention of mental disorders effective interventions and substance abuse in collaboration with the Prevention Research Center of the Universities of Nijmegen & Maastricht. Geneva (Switzerland): World Health Organization; 2004. p. 15.

48. Mrazek P, Haggerty R. Reducing risks for mental disorders: frontiers for preventive intervention research. Washington, DC: National Academy Press; 1994.

49. Detels R, McEwen J, Beaglehole R, et al. Oxford textbook of public health. 3rd edition. Oxford (UK): Oxford University Press; 2002.

50. World Health Organization. The Jakarta declaration on leading health promotion into the 21st Century. Geneva (Switzerland): World Health Organization; 1997.

51. Hosman C, Jane-Llopis E. Political challenges 2: mental health. In: Evidence of Health Promotion Effectiveness: Shaping Public Health in a New Europe. International Union for Health Promotion and Education (IUHPE). Paris: Jouve Composition & Impression 1999. p. 29–41. Chapter 3.

52. Patel V. Poverty, inequality and mental health in developing countries. In: Leon D, Walt G, editors. Poverty, inequality, and health. Oxford (UK): Oxford University Press; 2001. p. 247–62.

53. Grigg M, Hughes F. Role of nurses in mental health policy and planning: Australia and New Zealand. In: World Health Organization. Atlas: nurses in mental health. Geneva (Switzerland): WHO; 2007. p. 41.

54. Siantzde Leon ML. Leading change in diversity and cultural competence. J Prof Nurs 2008;24(3):167–71.

55. American Association of Colleges of Nursing. AACN position statement on the practice doctorate in nursing. Washington, DC: American Association of Colleges of Nursing; 2004.
56. Sheer B, Wong F. The development of advanced nursing practice globally. J Nurs Scholarsh 2008;40(3):201–11.
57. Villar Luis MA, Gray G. Mental health curriculum in nursing education. In: World Health Organization. Atlas: nurses in mental health. Geneva (Switzerland): WHO; 2007. p. 27.

Prevention Approaches in Child Mental Health Disorders

Kathleen R. Delaney, PhD, RN, PMH-NP[a],*,
Ruth "Topsy" Staten, PhD, RN, PMH-CNS[b]

KEYWORDS

- Prevention • Child mental health • Psychiatric nurses
- Selected interventions • Indicated interventions
- Mental health intervention

We all aspire for children to reach early school years trusting adults, having a sense of initiative, and a level of self-regulation such that they might master the challenges they face. Children deserve adults who are committed to providing the type of environments and relationships that support their progress toward these developmental milestones. Indeed, researchers have demonstrated such maturation occurs when children's surroundings are populated by reliable, responsive adults who support and when needed, augment their maturing cognitive and emotional regulation skills.[1,2] Now, via neuroscience, it is increasingly understood how these early environments, relationships, and experiences affect the developing brain and maturation.[3–5] Of particular interest are neural circuits that appear to mature and modify as information/experiences are presented to the developing infant, events the infant is primed to take in, process, and store.[4]

This perspective of experience-dependent development lends an expanded perspective on prevention and promotion. With increasing clarity, researchers understand how adults in the child's surroundings might intervene early to modify the environment or experiences so as to promote mental health and, in this process, actually prevent emotional or behavioral disorders.[6,7] With the knowledge that one-half of persons who experience mental health problems have symptoms before age 14 years and three-fourths by age 24,[8] clinicians who work with children and families must engage in critical opportunities to promote mental health and prevent development

[a] Department of Community, Systems and Mental Health Nursing, Rush College of Nursing, 600 South Paulina Street, Chicago, IL 60612, USA
[b] University of Kentucky, College of Nursing, 525 College of Nursing, Lexington, KY 40536-0232, USA
* Corresponding author.
E-mail address: Kathleen_R_Delaney@rush.edu

Nurs Clin N Am 45 (2010) 521–539
doi:10.1016/j.cnur.2010.06.002
0029-6465/10/$ – see front matter © 2010 Elsevier Inc. All rights reserved.

of advanced mental disorders in children who show early symptoms.[7] In the traditional disease model of illness care, one might simply wait until illness or at least a high level of symptoms appear, and then treat. This approach in the case of mental illness is costly not only in money and resources but also in the cost to human suffering, both for the person who is ill and his or her family.[6]

The newly released Institute of Medicine (IOM) Report, "Preventing mental, emotional and behavioral disorders among young people: progress and possibilities"[6] provides a road map for mental health promotion and mental health prevention. It is certainly the most current compendium of mental health promotion/prevention strategies. The IOM prevention approach is grounded in the complex interplay of genes, environment, risk, and protective factors that influence the manifestation of behavior. The focus of this article is on one aspect of the IOM initiative: prevention efforts aimed at processes thought to be involved in the development of mental illnesses. Readers should not lose sight that the development of a diagnosable mental illness is influenced by multiple factors operating as the child (with a particular set of risks and protective factors) moves through maturation and adapts to the environment.[9] The goal of the authors is to provide a resource on mental illness prevention for nurses who work with children, so the article begins with an overview of the IOM prevention paradigm and the levels of prevention.

A COMPREHENSIVE MODEL OF PREVENTION: EMPHASIS ON MENTAL HEALTH AND WELL-BEING

Organizations worldwide are calling for a public health approach to mental health promotion and mental illness prevention.[6,10–13] The prominence of mental health promotion and prevention represents a conceptual shift in the development and implementation of mental health interventions. Up to now, the emphasis has been on early recognition of symptoms and efforts to limit the impact of these symptoms on high-risk individuals.[7] Prevention activities were often focused on reducing the likelihood of disability or relapse for those individuals diagnosed with a mental disorder. Now, as explained in the IOM report,[6] prevention should focus on strategies that reduce risk before the onset of an identifiable mental disorder. Within this framework there are 3 levels of intervention: universal—general population; selective—at-risk individuals or populations; and indicated—at-risk individuals or populations who are experiencing minimal, but detectable signs or symptoms without meeting the diagnostic criteria (**Box 1**).

In this paradigm, the scope of mental health promotion broadens; that is, mental health is more than the absence of mental illness. According to the World Health Organization (WHO),[11] mental health is defined as "a state of well-being in which the individual realizes his or her own abilities, can cope with the normal stresses of life, can work productively and fruitfully, and is able to make a contribution to his or her community." For children, mental health and well-being include mastery of well-known challenges, that is, development of a sense of autonomy, industry, and initiative. Children's mental health also includes the development of capacities to form positive and helpful relationships, interact meaningfully with the environment, engage in self-regulation, and cope with adversity and challenges.[6]

Universal

Universal approaches to mental health promotion aim at assuring all children have healthy, supportive relationships and a safe/secure community environment. Of course, the broader social and economic environment also influences a child's mental

---

Box 1
Mental health promotion and mental illness prevention

Definitions and Programs

Mental Health Promotion: Interventions directed at the general public to enhance developmental competencies (task), a positive sense of self-esteem, mastery, and social connection, and to strengthen coping with adversity. Example: individual, school, and community programs that assure parents have positive mental health and skills to support children's development of social, emotional, and behavioral competencies.

Universal Prevention: Interventions targeted to whole population and not based on risk. Prevention efforts do focus on enhancement of protective factors against development of mental disorders. Example: School-based programs that teach coping skills or substance abuse resistance.

Selective Prevention: Interventions targeted at individuals or groups that are at risk of developing a mental health disorder, in the immediate or near future. Risk characteristics can be social, psychological, biologic, or economic. Examples: interventions offered to children and families with a destabilizing event such as divorce or parent absence.

Indicated Prevention: Interventions offered to individuals who are at risk of developing a mental disorder. These individuals may have minimal but detectable symptoms of a mental disorder but do not meet any disorder diagnostic criteria. Examples: interventions to reduce aggression, depressive symptoms, or elevated levels of anxiety.

Adapted from Institute of Medicine. Preventing mental, emotional, and behavioral disorders among young people: progress and possibilities. 2009. Available at: http://www.iom. edu/en/Reports/2009/Preventing-Mental-Emotional-and-Behavioral-Disorders-Among-Young-People-Progress-and-Possibilities.aspx. 2009; with permission.

---

health. Although public policy and funding are essential elements for a total approach to mental health promotion in children, discussion of these issues is beyond the scope of this article. Advocacy and policy work in prevention, however, should remain a priority for nurses who work to support children's mental health.

On a more immediate level, there are numerous opportunities for mental health promotion within reach of nurses who work with children and their families. Early environments and interaction with caregiving adults and parents is critical to healthy social-emotion-behavioral development and thus the well-being of children.[6] Mental health promotion of children begins with assuring that parents themselves are able to provide a loving relationship and an environment that supports critical relational, emotional, and behavioral developmental milestones.[6,10,11] In the next section the authors focus on 3 aspects of mental health promotion related to early relationships, all highly applicable to nurses who care for children, and all critical to development in children: (1) the screening, identification, and treatment of parents with emotional disorders; (2) infant and early childhood parenting practices; and (3) early childhood day care and education.

Screening, Evaluation, and Interventions for Parents

Adverse childhood events impact on an individual's mental and physical health, even long into adulthood.[14] One approach to prevention of adverse events is early recognition and treatment of mental, social, and behavioral problems in parents. Millions of adults in the United States, many of whom are parents, experience depression; but the effect of their depression on parenting and children's well-being is often ignored.[15] Evidence supports the benefits of depression screening in primary care,[15] but to date screening is still not routine. Despite the US Preventative Services Taskforce guidelines,[16] except in perinatal settings rarely does screening consider whether the adult is a parent or caregiver of young children. Screenings should be followed with evaluation, assessment of treatment options and preference, and care planning; yet this is not part of the screening routine in many settings. Screening often fails to include assessment for common comorbid disorders including anxiety and substance abuse disorders. Finally, screenings often fail to include the father,[15] even through a father's depression is linked to negative outcomes in the child, and even though researchers are finding significant levels of depressive symptoms in fathers, especially in families where there is maternal depression.[17,18]

The best outcomes for families are supported by universal screening in primary care and other community settings, particularly when followed by indicted evaluations and appropriate treatment. Considering the impact of a parent's depression on a child, nurses need to ensure that several critical screening recommendations are followed:

- Full implementation of the depression screening guidelines for primary care including assessment of comorbid disorders, and follow-up education and treatment.[16] Research indicates that the use of screening tools or 2 key screening questions provides better recognition than inconsistent, nonspecific, global clinical impressions. The 2 key screening questions are: (1) During the past month have you often been bothered by feeling down, depressed, or hopeless? (2) During the past month have you often been bothered by little interest or pleasure in doing things?[19]
- Integration of parental screening in child well checks and developmental assessments at pediatric clinics. The only time parents may see a health care provider or child guidance expert is when they take their children for a routine visit or an assessment. The American Academy of Pediatrics (AAP)[20] recommends 3 time periods for screening of language and social delays in childhood. Although the AAP does not mention maternal screening for depression at these evaluations, nurses should be alert for any signs of parental distress during developmental assessments because maternal depression is linked to development delays in their offspring.
- Screening in nontraditional settings. Nurses should initiate depression screening in other settings, particularly those where mothers who are at high risk for depression, such as homeless shelters and substance abuse treatment programs. Particular success has been realized with screening at in-home visitation programs for young, low-income mothers. Such programs that offer screening for depressive symptoms and evidence-based protocols for follow-up are effective in reducing the likelihood of parental depression and subsequent effects on children (**Box 2**).[21]

Treatment of the parents is prevention for their child. Nurses, by virtue of their presence in many traditional and nontraditional settings, have the opportunity to advocate a more inclusive and comprehensive approach to screening, referral, and engagement in treatment.

Supporting Maternal Sensitivity and Attachment

Secure maternal/infants attachments are built on sensitive and consistent responsiveness.[5] A large body of evidence supports the importance of the mother's ability to read and respond to her baby's signals as the infant moves from helplessness to mastery of developmental competencies.[2] This parental connectedness also provides for the necessary experiences whereby infants learn to react and regulate physiologic

---

Box 2
Reducing depressive symptoms in parents

The IOM reports[6,15] indicate that one of the most important emphases in children's mental health promotion and mental illness prevention is recognition and intervention for parental mental health, particularly depressive symptoms/disorders. Based on the principles of cognitive-behavioral therapy used in treating depression in women,[22] Peden and colleagues[21] tested an intervention focused on reducing depressive symptoms, negative thinking, and chronic stressors in low-income single mothers with young children. The intervention, delivered in 6 1-hour or 4 90-minute group sessions, taught the participants how to reduce negative thinking using thought-stopping techniques (STOP) and affirmations. Mothers were taught to recognize problematic or negative thoughts, use the STOP technique to disrupt the negative thoughts, and practice thought substitution to replace negative thoughts with positive affirmations. The strategies were practiced and reinforced through homework assignments. Participants who received the intervention reported greater reduction in negative thinking, chronic stressors, and depressive symptoms than the control group. Reduction in mothers' negative thinking also led to improved perceptions of their children's behaviors.[23]

---

arousal, emotions, and attention. Moreover, these secure relationships support the neural circuitry development that leads to self-regulation as well as the ability to develop healthy relationships and to respond effectively to unfamiliar and stressful situations[6]— a foundation for social, emotional, and behavioral competence throughout life.[24,25]

Promotion activities are successful in nurturing these positive parent-infant relationships. Yet there has been little investment in developing training or educational programs that support positive parenting practices in nonclinical parent populations.[26] The majority of the promotion research on supporting maternal sensitivity and attachment has been conducted with at-risk groups such as foster and adoptive families. In a review of these programs, Dozier[27] concluded that promising programs, ones that have the most enduring impact, share several features: they are time-limited, use brief interventions, target a specific aspect of parent interaction (such as increasing sensitivity), and begin during the second 6 months of an infant's life.

One of the most studied and successful programs aimed at mental health promotion and mental illness prevention in children is the David Olds Nurse Home Visiting Model (Nurse-Family Partnership).[28] Olds and colleagues recruited nurses to visit first-time, low-income single mothers from the prenatal period until the child was 2 years old. The program showed improvement in several areas; pregnancy outcomes, reduction in maternal substance abuse, mental health problems, and child abuse, and reduction in behavioral problems and criminal activities among the children.[29] In addition, mothers became more self-sufficient and children performed better in school.

The importance of fathers in the development of attachment has received little attention. It is well recognized that positive relationships with father's support healthy social-emotional development in children.[30] However, there has been little research into the development of programs that support fathers' interactions with children. Efforts in Canada serve as a prototype for the research that will eventually support promotion activities aimed at father's involvement.[31]

Early Childhood Day Care and Education

Day care settings and schools are also influential in shaping children's social, emotional, and behavioral development. Preschool programs such as Head Start that support social-emotional competence in children show gains not only in these areas but also improvements in academic success, enhanced school-parent relationships, and reduced external and internalizing disorders in children.[32] Nurses who work with high-risk toddlers should encourage parents toward these programs, educating them on the potential of these programs to boost children's social-emotional competencies; skills that have broad benefits for the child's future.

Day care and preschool programs may also provide resources that enhance the home environment and classroom. The Incredible Years Program (IPY), a universal and targeted prevention program, includes components for family/parent, child, and school/teacher.[33] IPY has universal outcomes of strengthening all students' social-emotional competence, increasing self-control behaviors, and reducing aggression and associated behaviors in children who are exhibiting problems. Building on the strong evidence base of the IPY program, Gross and colleagues[34] adapted the protocol for, and in collaboration with, African American and Latino families in Chicago (**Box 3**). Early testing of their program indicates that it succeeded in designing a culturally sensitive intervention that promoted positive parenting and effective discipline strategies.

MOVING THE PREVENTION PARADIGM FORWARD: NURSES' ROLE IN SELECTIVE AND INDICATED INTERVENTIONS

The IOM report[6] isolated several areas of particular relevance to nurses: early intervention with at-risk young mothers, parenting programs, and prevention programs that target specific disorders.[35] There is certainly much in this report for nurses, particularly as they move within their clinical sites toward the goal of a prevention-oriented mental health system of care for children.[36–38] For example, school nurses will likely be participating in whole school efforts to build positive youth development programs, perhaps via the development of a social-emotional learning culture.[39] Pediatric nurses practicing in community settings will soon have opportunities to participate in the primary care initiatives aimed at early identification of and intervention in common mental health issues.[40]

The challenge for nurses is to recognize the multiple levels of promotion and thus the multiple opportunities that their direct care positions afford to intervene and prevent the progression of mental illness. Indeed, prevention research should inform the daily practice of nurses who work with children. This group is the large cohort of nurses practicing in schools, hospitals, communities, and specialty areas such as juvenile

---

Box 3
Behavioral parent training: the Chicago parent project

The IOM report cites Behavioral Parent Training (BPT) as an evidence-based prevention that is especially useful for parents dealing with children who are difficult to manage. One of the most widely distributed BPT programs is the Incredible Years BASIC (IYP) program developed by Carolyn Webster-Stratton, which uses group discussion of videotaped parent-child interactions to develop parent's problem solving, positive parenting approaches, and effective limit setting. The program has demonstrated success at increasing parent's self efficacy at handling difficult behaviors and also reducing children's behavior problems.[33] The Chicago Parent Program builds on the methods of IYP but, recognizing its inconsistent outcomes with ethnic minority preschool children, revised the parent discussion vignettes in consultation with an advisory board of African American and Latino parents. These new videotaped scenes were more compatible with the challenges these parents face, and suggested parenting strategies they considered congruent with their values and culture.[34] These videotaped vignettes were used in a trial of the program across 7 day care centers; 4 were initially allocated to wait-list control but in 2004 also became intervention centers. The intervention was effective in reducing corporal punishment and the number of parental commands. Child behavior problems also declined. The positive effects of the intervention were greatest among the group of parents who attended the most sessions.[34] In discussion of results, the researchers highlight how they incorporated culturally sensitive approaches to issues such as spanking, and how their program successful adapted preventive parent training to low-income African American and Latino parents.

justice. The challenge is viewed as isolating threads of prevention research and practice such that it becomes useable to nurses who have direct involvement with children and their families.

In addition to universal prevention, nurses should consider how to bring selective and indicated prevention interventions into their workplaces, particularly those aimed at specific disorders thought to make an appearance during childhood. Indicated and selective prevention efforts can be seen to target the causal pathways that lead to mental, emotional, and behavioral (MEB) problems.[30] In this view, there is particular emphasis on the neurobiological underpinnings of particular MEB disorders, on maintaining that select disorders take root in dynamic disruptions in key developmental processes, and on disruptions that continue to effect maturation and positive adoption throughout the life span.[6] For instance, while attachment has long been recognized as vital to mental health, there is increasing interest in the specific experience-dependent synaptic growth that occurs with attachment experiences; that is, synaptic growth which ushers in greater connectivity of the prefrontal areas (thinking and planning) and limbic (emotional) structures.[41] This connectivity provides the platform for emotional regulation that relies on, among others, the ability to think or objectify what one is feeling.[4] Thus prevention efforts aimed at populations at risk for attachment derailments might also be intervening at the very start of emotional regulation problems; regulation issues which, if left unchecked, can be tied to any number of psychopathologies in children.[42] With the mutual progress of neuroscience and intervention research, each informing the other, the horizon of selective prevention broadens.

The synergy of prevention and developmental neuroscience is progressing, particularly in the context of 3 specific childhood disorders: anxiety, depression, and disruptive behavior disorders. The particular interest here is on prevention interventions that target processes thought to drive psychological processes relevant to the origins of these mental illnesses.[43] For each disorder, discussion includes the emerging prevention science, particular evidence-based selective interventions, and suggestions for applying this knowledge in nursing practice with children and families.

To create prevention-oriented systems of care for children, the practice of prevention cannot be isolated to manualized programs. Rather, clinicians should integrate principles of prevention as they work with families to build regulation and resilience in children displaying identified risk behaviors.[44] To help us reach this goal, there needs to be a bridge for bringing selective and indicated prevention focus into the everyday practice of direct care practitioners. The authors suggest that one way to build this bridge is mapping how prevention foci address psychological processes thought to be involved in particular mental illnesses. It is proposed that grasping prevention science from this angle will help nurses bridge across the science and integrate prevention-oriented approaches into their practice.

Anxiety Disorders

Healthy development starts in the prenatal environment, and it is well documented that mental health promotion and prevention is vital at this stage as well as in early infancy.[7] Interest is focused on the school-age child who is involved with developmental tasks around school performance and peer relationships because it is a period of demands that require the child to self-regulate emotions and behaviors, including negative emotions such as anxiety and distress.[45] Anxiety in children is one of the most pervasive of childhood disorders, affecting 10% to 15% of children,[46] and the accompanying worry, apprehension, fear, and distress can significantly interfere with developmental demands. If left untreated, anxiety can become a risk factor for several negative sequelae including the development of other serious emotional disorders such as depression.[47] The types of anxiety are as varied as is the underlying neurobiology.[48] Therefore, the focus here is on the group of anxiety disorders that begin to appear in childhood (separation anxiety disorder, social phobia, and generalized anxiety disorder)[49] and the secondary prevention efforts that address modifiable factors: parent/family factors (such as overprotection) and the child's anxiety/avoidant symptoms and maladaptive cognitions.[50,51]

In a series of studies, Kagan and colleagues[52] demonstrated that particular children are born with inhibited temperaments. Now scientists believe that inhibited behaviors may go beyond shy temperament and that such children may be more likely to progress into the anxiety spectrum.[49,53] Viewing shy temperament as a risk factor for anxiety disorders provides a theoretical platform for preventive interventions targeted to young, inhibited children.[54] One such prevention program designed for pre–school-age children centers on parental education. In this program parents learn about the nature of anxiety, how overprotection might maintain anxiety, and incorporates principles of exposure and cognitive restructuring.[55] Outcomes indicated that although this parental education intervention did not have an impact on the child's temperament, it did reduce the number of anxiety disorders in children 12 months after intervention. This type of intervention fits into the nursing paradigm of family involvement because, via education, the parent becomes the interventionist, working to modify behaviors that may increase anxiety in a child at risk.

Another approach to secondary prevention of childhood anxiety disorders targets parents who have a diagnosed anxiety disorder. Having a parent with an anxiety disorder is considered a significant risk factor for the child[56]; a familial risk that may involve more than genes. Researchers suggest that anxious parents shape the social information processing templates of their children by reinforcing attention to threat and legitimizing apprehension.[57] A secondary prevention project that targeted families enrolled parents who had a current or lifetime diagnosis of anxiety and a child between the ages 7 and 12.[58] The program was designed to address several modifiable risk factors, teaching parents how to reduce parental overprotection and how to avoid modeling anxious responses. It also presented instruction on cognitive restructuring and building children's problem-solving skills. Via this program, Ginsburg[58] successfully reduced the expression of anxiety symptoms in children in the treatment group.

Several secondary prevention programs are also tailored to children who are exhibiting anxiety behaviors. Several of these studies use a Cognitive Behavioral Treatment (CBT) framework, akin to the Kendall's successful treatment program.[59] The premise of this CBT model is that children exhibiting early signs of anxiety have a pattern of fearful responses to particular stimuli that affects how they pay attention to the event and attributions they form about the cause of the event.[60] The child may also have vulnerability for fearful responses to even benign stimuli. The critical factor is that the repeated experiences of apprehension establish a cognitive template (or filter), which then begins to influence how the child allocates attention, that is, they have difficulty switching focus away from anxiety-provoking events.[49] In the CBT framework the child learns first to recognize anxious feelings, then examines the accompanying attributions, and finally practices alternative ways of thinking about the situation.[61] In a sense, with this reappraisal of anxious thoughts the child is building a new, more adaptive cognitive template around particular events.

Such a strategy is at the heart of selective prevention intervention studies conducted largely in Australia. In each of the studies[62,63] investigators intervened with school-age children displaying anxious behaviors. The program involved education about anxiety, cognitive restructuring techniques, gradual exposure, and skill-building modules. In each study the children in the treatment group displayed a reduction in anxiety behaviors, and in one of the studies, gains were evident 2 years after intervention.[62] Replication of this program in the United States with children displaying mild to moderate anxiety symptoms also resulted in significant reduction in children's anxiety symptoms post intervention.[64]

How can nurses use this information about successful selective prevention efforts? Of course, if such prevention programs are available in the community, nurses might refer children deemed to be at risk. Nurses can also integrate a prevention approach into their practice by drawing on the content/process of efficacious selective interventions, particularly how the interventions address key psychological processes thought to be fundamental to the progression of anxiety disorders. As outlined here, several of the interventions used a CBT framework that aimed to dampen a child's anxious response by both identifying the emotion and challenging fearful/catastrophic thoughts. Theoretically, such an approach enhances the cortical processing circuits that interpret stimuli, which in turn dampen subcortical (amygdala) activation.[65] For example, an imaging study specific to CBT treatments for social phobia with adults indicated that following therapy, when faced with an anxiety-provoking task, those in the treatment group demonstrated a reduction in amygdala activation.[66]

Particularly important for nurses in practice is their understanding of the rationale for interventions involving parents. Overattention by anxious children to threat in the environment is a key psychological process of their disorders,[67–69] and emerging neuroscience suggests that reducing attention to threat is a critical element in addressing emotional regulation issues.[70,71] Parental overprotection of anxious children has several untoward effects, one being that anxious parents may reinforce attention to threat.[57] Teaching parents about the relationship of anxiety and threat attention would be a useful platform for examining the issue of overprotection. Thus nurses might integrate secondary prevention science into practice as they themselves come to understand and then teach families why CBT dampens anxious associations, why threat orientation/appraisal is a key component of anxiety, and finally why with early intervention children might begin to retrain how they allocate attention.[49]

Depression: Early Prevention

As outlined in the IOM[6] report, much of the prevention efforts aimed at depression have targeted adolescents. In a review of depression prevention efforts, 7 of which targeted adolescents, Cuijpers and colleagues[72] concluded that prevention can check the appearance of new depressive disorders in adolescents, particularly with those teens displaying more depressive symptoms. In a review of depression prevention studies that compared the effect sizes of interventions, the results of child prevention efforts were less promising then several implemented with adolescents.[73] In this meta-analysis, Horowitz and Garber questioned if the majority of the studies they reviewed were true prevention interventions. The investigators noted that only 4 of the 30 studies reviewed reported elevated depression scores of the control group, whereas there was no increase in scores for the treatment group. Thus they argue that much of the selective/indicated prevention programs, which often report outcomes as a decrease of depressive symptoms in the intervention group, should be categorized as treatment of early depression.

Whether for early treatment or prevention, it is important to address depressive symptoms as soon as they become evident because of the serious ramifications of depression in youth.[74] In reviews of depression treatment programs for children and adolescents, 2 secondary prevention programs designed for children were identified as probably efficacious: the Penn Prevention Program (also known as the Penn Resiliency Program) and programs based on Self Control Theory.[75,76] These 2 programs are examined here, with a particular focus on isolating why (theoretically) the intervention should dampen depressive symptoms. Recently, Miller[77] suggested that there are several fundamental components to depression: hedonic capacity, stress sensitivity, and ruminative self-focus. Using this framework, one might frame selective/indicated prevention interventions according to how they address one of these fundamental components, that is, how prevention speaks to a child's loss of interest and lack of pleasure (hedonic capacity), how they boost resilience in response to stress-provoking events, or how prevention efforts intervene at the level of a child's ruminative negative self-focus.

A prevention program for middle school-age youth that aims at improving both response to stress and negative self-focus is the Penn Resiliency Program.[78] In this program preadolescents are taught the linkages between how they think, feel, and behave, as well as problem-solving skills. Using a CBT approach, they are also taught how to challenge negative thinking: evaluate the accuracy of the thought and the evidence to support it, and then devise an alternative, more positive response. This program has been implemented in a variety of settings, including schools[79] and primary care.[80] In a summary of the program's outcomes across 13 studies, Gillham and Reivich[81] recognized there have been some inconsistent findings, but maintain the data demonstrate that the intervention prevents symptoms of anxiety and depression. Although there has been some question of its effectiveness with culturally diverse populations, a variation has been successfully implemented with children of Chinese descent[82] and it has produced positive outcomes with Latino children.[83] When the program was implemented in a study in Australia, the findings supported positive changes in the participants' anxiety levels and with helping them build a more optimistic explanatory style.[84]

Another promising efficacious secondary prevention program, identified by the acronym ACTION, is based on self-control therapy.[85] This program teaches children how to recognize emotions, particularly negative moods, and thus become more aware of their moods and responses. Children also learn how to use strategies such as problem solving or cognitive restructuring to address their negative emotions and cognitions. Via these strategies children find that they can deal with negative moods and experiences, which builds their sense of control and confidence so that they can take action to improve their mood. Variations of the program have been tested with diverse populations.[86] Depressed youth often view stressful events as overwhelming; thus instilling a perception that provokes a hopeless response.[87] By empowering youth to deal with stress, ACTION addresses a fundamental component of youth depression.

Another widely used approach for secondary prevention with school-age children targets parents who are dealing with depression. For over 2 decades it has been recognized that parents' depression affects their children in a variety of ways, including adjustment problems, emotional issues, and clinical depression.[15,88,89] The relationship of child regulation issues and parental depression has been studied from a variety of approaches. For instance, research has demonstrated that children who have a tendency toward aggressive/anger behaviors who are raised by a depressed mother show a greater tendency toward aggression, anxiety, and depression.[90] In another study the children of depressed mothers, particularly those with marked behavioral inhibition, were shown to have significant issues with emotional regulation, principally the upregulation of negative emotions.[91] Children raised by depressed mothers, especially girls, have been shown to exhibit a more passive style of regulating emotion, and have difficultly shifting attention from distressing stimuli.[92] Thus maternal depression seems to have an impact on their offspring's emotional regulation competence, particularly in the area of suppressing negative emotions and regulating aggression/anger.

Considering its impact on children and the long-standing awareness of its effects, it is not surprising that parental depression has been a focus of prevention efforts for over 15 years. A recent review examined the outcomes of these programs and the association between improvement in parental depression and decreases in child psychopathology.[93] In sum, the 10 studies reviewed demonstrated a relationship between successful treatment of parental depression and improvement in children's symptoms and functioning. Awareness of the wide-ranging impact of maternal depression and of the benefits of dealing with the problem should motivate nurses to address this sensitive topic of parents' mental health issues.

Finally, in a unique approach, a successful selective prevention program intervenes directly with the children of depressed parent.[94] Aiming to build resiliency in children, affect predepression symptoms, and nurture a shared family understanding, the researchers teach children about their parents' illness. Parents learn about how to talk about their illness with their children. In several studies the researchers demonstrated that their intervention increased children's understanding of their parents' illness and that the children's internalizing symptomatology decreased.[84,95] In follow-up studies with a large portion of the original sample, the investigators found that children's gains in understanding their parents' illness were sustained, as was a reduction in internalizing symptoms.[96] This intervention is seen to boost youth resiliency because it provides youth with the tools to build resources necessary to thrive in what might be considered an environment that puts them at risk.[95]

When nurses encounter a child displaying depressive symptoms, the most straightforward secondary prevention intervention is to refer the child and his or her family to a program tailored to their risk behaviors. Understanding the elements of these programs should inform nurses on the basic platform of prevention efforts in depression. As evidenced by these prevention programs, children can be taught how to challenge negative thinking with more adaptive responses. It also seems possible to increase children's awareness of their negative moods and empower them to change the situation generating the distress. Finally, it is possible to teach problem-solving skills so that children will have additional tools for dealing with stress. Considering the negative effects of maternal depression on the offspring, nurses must be alert to and discuss with parents any apparent signs and symptoms of their distress. Knowledge of prevention research will increase nurses' ability to enter into this delicate interpersonal territory. Along with educating parents on how their illness may have an effect on their child, nurses might also point out the importance of building the child's understanding of the illness to buffer the impact. Indeed nurses must tread a careful line to avoid what might be interpreted as critical, an approach that only increases stigma.[97] By framing the conversation in the emerging science of prevention, nurses decrease any hint of blame and build a sense of partnership with parents around building their child' resiliency.

Disruptive Behavior Disorders

Disruptive behavior problems (DBP) in children manifest as noncompliance, aggression, and negative emotionality. Although a DSM-IV (*Diagnostic and Statistical Manual of Mental Disorders* Fourth Edition) diagnosis, a degree of controversy surrounds the DBP classification, particularly when the criteria are applied to preschool children.[98] Yet as assessment tools are developed specific to DBP, it has become clear that symptoms of DBP can be isolated and that screening tools do differentiate youth referred for problem behavior from nonreferred preschool children.[98,99] Because aggression and noncompliance of young children are frequent issues both in pediatric primary care and mental health clinics, it is important that nurses who deal with children understand the boundaries of the disorder and the basis for prevention efforts.[100]

In the IOM prevention scheme,[6] behaviors that are usually considered under the category of DBP are introduced as issues of family disruption, not as a specific mental/emotional/behavioral presentation. In line with framing the issue as one of family disruption, the IOM report[6] highlights several selective prevention programs designed for family intervention. The report takes particular note of BPT, a variation of which is highlighted earlier in the article (see **Box 2**). Because there are many variations of BPT, nurses should be aware of the basic prevention process involved in such training, that is, how the intervention aims at building parenting skills particularly for families dealing with a child who is difficult to manage.[101,102]

Several universal school-based programs aim at the prevention of behavior problems in youth. Such programs are generally structured around building positive school environments that support both effective problem solving and systems of rules and consequences.[103] Nurses' interest is on the functional components of selective and indicated prevention programs and how nurses might use these data to inform their work. In this light the authors consider a secondary prevention program that has addressed children deemed at risk for DBP, The Fast Track Program (Conduct prevention) implementing the PATHS curriculum (Promoting Alternative Thinking Strategies).[104] When implemented with high-risk populations, PATHS seeks to enhance the social-emotional competencies of children.

The program emphasizes the relationship between emotion, cognition, language, and behavior, and includes interventions that help children recognize emotions, initiate problem solving in the context of specific situations, and learn strategies for conscious self-control.[105] In a multisite test of the program, children in the intervention group showed progress in these social-emotional skills and also demonstrated improvements in peer relationships and language arts grades.[106] Recently, the Conduct Problems Prevention Group[107] tested if the outcomes of the intervention changed in children who varied in their level of initial risk. Looking at a cohort 10 years after intervention, the greatest effects were with children that were initially deemed at high risk. These children now displayed significantly less externalizing disorders. Thus the PATHS curriculum, which aims to build emotional regulation and executive functions, is also successful at decreasing the expression of conduct-like disorders.

The Prevention Group also explored exactly how the PATHS intervention works, that is, what specific aspects of social-emotional functioning and neurocognitive capacity the model addresses.[108] The researchers proposed that the PATHS model decreased the expression of conduct-like disorders because it improved children's executive function and verbal fluency, particularly the ability to talk about effects and situations. Executive functions are a group of cognitively mediated skills such as attention shifting and planning. These skills help the child inhibit their initial (perhaps impulsive) reaction and direct attention to a response that might help them successfully address the personal, situational, or interpersonal task demands that confront them.[108] The researchers used neurocognitive testing and determined that several of the positive gains (decreased externalizing/internalizing behaviors) in the intervention group could be explained by their progress with inhibitory control or verbal fluency.[108] These data are extremely useful for nurses who often see parents dealing with their young child's noncompliance or anger/aggression. BPT is an effective intervention for these issues, particularly if parents enlist help early in preschool years. School-age children who are displaying aggression or negative behaviors might be referred to a prevention program available within the child's school. But nurses can also help parents use the basic elements of such programs as the PATHS model, that is, teaching children strategies for self-control and emotional recognition/regulation skills. These types of interventions map how children ultimately develop effortful control, the conscious control of thought, or ability to direct attention or suppress initial reactions in the service of longer term goals.[109] This is essential science for nurses working with young children and their parents; it holds useful connections between emotion-based early intervention and the development of regulation skills.[110]

SUMMARY

Mental health promotion and mental illness prevention research hold much promise for the healthy development and well-being of our children. The expanded vision of prevention brings with it guidance for how front-line clinicians might partner with families and schools to build protective processes that will help children develop social-emotional competence and cope with challenges, be it a parent struggling with depression or a trait of high emotional reactivity. Nurses, with the vast array of roles and settings in which they interact with families, parents, and children, are in a unique position to promote health attachments, development of self-soothing and self-control behaviors, and prosocial, positive relationships. Increasingly for select serious emotional illnesses, the basics of particular selective and indicated prevention approaches can be mapped on the emerging neuroscience of the disorder. Nurses might also fit together prevention science with the promising models that link neural circuits, basic psychological processes, and illness phenotypes.[69] This disciplinary knowledge, along with prevention science, is a useful platform for nurses as they work with parents and children at risk for a serious emotional illness. Children develop regulation skills in a complex interplay of maturation and parental guidance. The urgency for early intervention grows as clinicians and parents understand how children might build protective processes that buffer vulnerabilities to regulation issues, and thus help them continue on a developmental trajectory to optimum mental health.

REFERENCES

1. Emde RN. Mobilizing fundamental modes of development. J Am Psychoanal Assoc 1990;38:889–913.
2. Stern DN. The interpersonal world of the infant. New York: Basic books; 1985.
3. Schore AN. Affect regulation and the repair of the self. New York: W.W. Norton; 2003.
4. Siegel DJ. The developing mind: how relationships and the brain interact to shape who we are. New York: Guilford Press; 1999.
5. Tryon WW. Cognitive processes in cognitive and psychological therapies. Cognitive The Res 2009;33:570–84.
6. Institute of Medicine. Preventing mental, emotional, and behavioral disorders among young people: progress and possibilities. 2009. Available at: http://www.iom.edu/en/Reports/2009/Preventing-Mental-Emotional-and-Behavioral-Disorders-Among-Young-People-Progress-and-Possibilities.aspx. Accessed September 1, 2009.
7. Mrazek PJ, Haggerty RJ. Reducing risks for mental disorders: frontiers for preventive intervention research. Washington, DC: National Academies Press; 1994.
8. Kessler RC, Berglund P, Demler O, et al. Lifetime prevalence and age-of-onset distributions of DSM-IV disorders in the national comorbidity survey replication. Arch Gen Psychiatry 2005;62:593–602.
9. Sroufe PL. Psychopathology as an outcome of development. Dev Psycopathol 1997;9:251–68.
10. Substance Abuse and Mental Health Services Administration, Center for Mental Health Services (SAMHSA). Promotion and prevention in mental

health: strengthening parenting and enhancing child resilience, DHHS Publication No. CMHS-SVP-0175. Rockville (MD); 2007.

11. World Health Organization. Prevention and promotion in mental health. Geneva (Switzerland): World health organization; 2002.

12. Cohen E, Kaufmann R. Early childhood mental health consultation. DHHS Pub. No. CMHS SVP0151. Rockville (MD): Center for Mental Health Services, Substance Abuse and Mental Health Services Administration; 2005.

13. New Freedom Commission on Mental Health, Achieving the promise: transforming mental health care in America. final report. DHHS Pub. No. SMA-03-3832. Rockville (MD); 2003.

14. Felliti V, Anda R, Nordenberg D, et al. Relationship of childhood abuse and household dysfunction to many of the leading causes of death in adults: the adverse childhood experiences (ACE) study. Am J Prev Med 1998;14(4): 246–58.

15. National Research Council and Institute of Medicine. Depression in parents, parenting, and children: opportunities to improve identification, treatment, and prevention. Committee on Depression, Parenting Practices, and the Healthy Development of Children. Board on Children, Youth, and Families. Washington, DC: The National Academies Press; 2009.

16. U.S. Preventative Services Taskforce (USPSTF) Guidelines. Screening for depression in adults: U.S. preventive services task force recommendation statement. Ann Intern Med 2009;151:784–92.

17. Ramchandani P, Stein A, Evans J, et al. Paternal depression in the postnatal period and child development: a prospective population study. Lancet 2005; 365(9478):2201–5.

18. Ramchandani P, Psychogiou L. Paternal psychiatric disorders and children's psychosocial development. Lancet 2009;374(9690):646–53.

19. Whooley MA, Avins AL, Miranda J, et al. Case finding instruments for depression: two questions as good as many. J Gen Intern Med 1997;12:439–45.

20. American Academy of Pediatrics and Council on Children with Disabilities. Identifying infants and young children with developmental disorders in the medical home: An algorithm for developmental surveillance and screening. Pediatrics 2006;118:405–20.

21. Peden A, Rayens MK, Hall L, et al. Testing an intervention to reduce negative thinking, depressive symptoms, and chronic stressors in low-income single mother. J Nurs Scholarsh 2005;37(3):268–74.

22. Gordon VC, Tobin M. Insight: a cognitive enhancement program for women. Available from. Minneapolis (MN): Verona Gordon, University of Minnesota; 1991.

23. Hall L, Rayens MK, Peden A. Maternal factors associated with child behavior. J Nurs Scholarsh 2008;40(2):124–30.

24. Bronson M. Self regulation in early childhood. New York: Guilford Press; 2002.

25. Brownell C, Kopp M. Socioemotional development in toddler years. New York: Guilford Press; 2007.

26. Ranson K, Urichuk L. The effect of parent-child attachment and relationships on child biopsychosocial outcomes: a review. Early Child Dev Care 2008;178(2): 129–52.

27. Dozier M. The impact of attachment-based interventions on the quality of attachment among infants and young children. In: Tremblay RE, Barr RG, Peters RDeV, editors. Encyclopedia on early childhood development. Montreal (QC): Centre of Excellence for Early Childhood Development; 2004. p. 1–5.

28. Nurse-Family Partnership History and Goals. Available at: http://www. nursefamilypartnership.org/index.cfm?fuseaction=home. Accessed December 12, 2009.
29. Olds DL, Hill PL, O'Brien R, et al. Taking preventive intervention to scale: the nurse-family partnership. Cogn Behav Pract 2003;10:278–90.
30. National Research Council and Institute of Medicine. From neurons to neighborhoods: the science of early childhood development. committee on integrating the science of early childhood development. In: Shonkoff JP, Phillips DA, editors. Board on children, youth, and families, commission on behavioral and social sciences and education. Washington (DC): National Academy Press; 2000.
31. Father Involvement Research Alliance (FIRA). FIRA vision, values and the future. Available at: http://www.fira.ca/page.php?id=8. Accessed December 12, 2009.
32. Love JM, Kisker EE, Ross CM, et al. Making a difference in the lives of infants and toddlers and their families: the impacts of early head start. I: final technical report. Princeton (NJ): Mathematica Policy Research; 2002.
33. Webster –Stratton C. Prevention conduct problems in Head Start children: strengthening parenting competencies. J Consult Clin Psychol 1998;66:715–30.
34. Gross D, Garvey C, Julion W, et al. Efficacy of the Chicago parent program with low-income African American and Latino parents of young children. Prev Sci 2009;10:54–65.
35. Evans ME. Prevention of mental, emotional, and behavioral disorders in Youth: The Institute of Medicine Report and implications for nursing. J Child Adolesc Psychiatr Nurs 2009;22:154–9.
36. Huang L, Macbeth G, Dodge J, et al. Transforming the workforce in children's mental health. Adm Policy Ment Health 2004;32:167–87.
37. National Association of Pediatric Nurse Practitioners. NAPNAP position statement of integration of mental health care in pediatric primary care settings. J Pediatr Health Care 2007;21:29A–30A.
38. Stephan SH, Weist M, Kataoka S, et al. Transformation of Children's mental health services: the role of school mental health. Psychiatr Serv 2007;58:1330–8.
39. Weissberg RP, O'Brien MU. What works in school-based social and emotional learning programs for positive youth development. Ann Am Acad Pol Soc Sci 2004;591:86–97.
40. American Academy of Pediatrics. Policy statement—the future of Pediatrics: mental health competencies for pediatric primary care. Pediatrics 2009;124: 410–21.
41. Schore A. The effects of early relational trauma on right brain development, affect regulation and infant mental health. Infant Mental Health J 2001;22: 201–69.
42. Fonagy P, Target M. Early intervention and the development of self-regulation. Psychoanal Inq 2002;22:307–35.
43. March JS. The future of psychotherapy for mentally ill children and adolescents. J Child Psychol Psychiatry 2009;10:170–9.
44. Delaney KR. Psychotherapy with children. In: Wheeler K, editor. Psychotherapy for the advanced practice nurse. St. Louis: Mosby; 2008. p. 330–5.
45. Masten AS, Coatsworth JD. The development of competence in favorable and unfavorable environments: lessons from research on successful children. Am Psychol 1998;53:205–20.
46. Costello EJ, Mustillo S, Erkanli A, et al. Prevalence and development of psychiatric disorders in childhood and adolescents. Arch Gen Psychiatry 2003;60: 837–44.

47. Cole DA, Peeke LG, Maring JM. A longitudinal look at the relation between depression and anxiety in children and adolescents. J Consult Clin Psychol 1998;66:451–60.

48. Engel K, Bandelow B, Gruber O. Neuroimaging in anxiety disorders. J Neural Transm 2009;116:703–16.

49. Pine DS. Research review: a neuroscience framework for pediatric anxiety disorders. J Child Psychol Psychiatry 2007;48:631–48.

50. Bienvenu OJ, Ginsburg GS. Prevention of anxiety disorders. Int Rev Psychiatry 2007;19:647–54.

51. Neil AL, Christensen H. Efficacy and effectiveness of school based prevention and early intervention programs for anxiety. Clin Psychol Rev 2009;29:208–15.

52. Kagan J, Reznick JS, Snidman N. Biological bases of childhood shyness. Science 1988;240:167–71.

53. Perez-Edgar K, Fox NA. Temperament and anxiety disorders. Child Adolesc Psychiatr Clin N Am 2005;14:681–706.

54. Rapee RM. The development and modification of temperamental risk for anxiety disorders: prevention of a lifetime of anxiety. Biol Psychiatry 2002;52:947–57.

55. Rapee RM, Kennedy S, Ingram M. Prevention and early intervention of anxiety disorders in inhibited preschool children. J Consult Clin Psychol 2005;73: 488–97.

56. Beidel DC, Turner SM. At risk for anxiety: I. Psychopathology in the offspring of anxious parents. J Am Acad Child Adolsec Psychiatry 1997;36:918–24.

57. Derryberry D, Reed MA. Regulatory processes and the development of cognitive representations. Dev Psychopathol 1996;8:215–34.

58. Ginsburg GS. The Child Anxiety Prevention Study: intervention model and primary outcomes. J Consult Clin Psychol 2009;77:580–7.

59. Kendall PC. Treatment of anxiety disorders in children: a randomized clinical trial. J Consult Clin Psychol 1994;62:100–10.

60. Kendall PC. Guiding theory for therapy with children and adolescents. In: Kendall PC, editor. Child and adolescent therapies: cognitive-behavioral procedures. 3rd edition. New York: Guilford Press; 2006. p. 3–31.

61. Kendall PC, Suveg C. Treating anxiety disorders in youth. In: Kendall PC, editor. Child and adolescent therapies: cognitive-behavioral procedures. 3rd edition. New York: Guilford Press; 2006. p. 243–94 REVIEW.

62. Dadds M, Holland DE, Spence SH. Early intervention and prevention of anxiety disorders in children: results of a 2 year follow-up. J Consult Clin Psychol 1999; 67:145–50.

63. Mifsud C, Rapee RM. Early intervention for childhood anxiety in a school setting: outcomes for an economically disadvantaged population. J Am Acad Child Adolesc Psychiatry 2005;44:996–1004.

64. Bernstein GA, Layne AE, Egan EA, et al. School-based interventions for anxious children. J Am Acad Child Adolesc Psychiatry 2005;44:1118–27.

65. Cozolino LJ. The neuroscience of psychotherapy. New York: W.W. Norton; 2002.

66. Porto PR, Oliveira L, Mari J, et al. Does cognitive behavioral therapy change the brain? A systematic review of neuroimaging in anxiety disorders. J Neuropsychiatry Clin Neurosci 2009;21:114–25.

67. Muris P, Meesters C, Rompelberg L. Attention control in middle childhood: relations to psychopathological symptoms and threat perception distortions. Behav Res Ther 2006;45:997–1010.

68. Roy AK, Vasa RA, Bruck M, et al. Attention bias toward threat in pediatric anxiety disorders. J Am Acad Child Adolesc Psychiatry 2008;47:1189–96.

69. Pine DS, Guyer AE, Leibenluft E. Functional Magnetic resonance imaging and pediatric anxiety. J Am Acad Child Adolesc Psychiatry 2008;47:1217–21.
70. Goldin PR, Manber T, Hakimi S. Neural bases of social anxiety disorder: emotional reactivity and cognitive regulation during social and physical play. Arch Gen Psychiatry 2009;66:170–80.
71. Oschsner KN, Gross JJ. Thinking makes it so: a social cognitive neuroscience approach to emotional regulation. In: Baumeister RF, Vohs KD, editors. Handbook of self regulation. New York: Guilford Press; 2004. p. 229–55.
72. Cuijpers P, Straten A, van Smit F, et al. Preventing the onset of depressive disorders: a meta-analytic review of psychological interventions. Am J Psychiatry 2008;165: 1272–80.
73. Horowitz JL, Garber J. The prevention of depressive symptoms in children and adolescents: a meta-analytic review. J Consult Clin Psychol 2006;74:401–15.
74. Foley DL, Goldston DB, Costello J. Proximal psychiatric risk factors for suicidality in youth. The Great Smokey Mountains Study. Arch Gen Psychiatry 2006;63:1017–24.
75. Greenberg MT, Domitrovich C, Bumbarger B. Preventing mental disorders in school aged children: a review of the effectiveness of prevention programs. Pennsylvania: Prevention Research Center for the Promotion of Human Development College of Health and Human Development Pennsylvania State University; 2000.
76. David-Ferdon C, Kaslow NJ. Evidence-based psychosocial treatments for child and adolescent depression. J Clin Child Adolesc Psychol 2008;37:62–104.
77. Miller A. Social neuroscience of child and adolescent depression. Brain Cogn 2007;65:47–68.
78. Penn resiliency project. Available at: http://www.ppc.sas.upenn.edu/prplessons.pdf. Accessed June 23, 2010.
79. Gillham JE, Reivich KJ, Freres DR. School-based prevention of depressive symptoms: a randomized controlled study of the effectiveness and specificity of the Penn Resiliency Program. J Consult Clin Psychol 2007;75:9–19.
80. Gillham JE, Hamilton J, Freres DR. Preventing depression among early adolescents in the primary care setting: a randomized controlled study of the Penn Resiliency Program. J Abnorm Child Psychol 2006;34:203–19.
81. Gillham JE, Reivich KJ. Resilience research in children. Available at: http://www.ppc.sas.upenn.edu/prpsum.htm. Accessed August 1, 2009.
82. Yu DL, Seligman ME. Preventing depressive symptoms in Chinese children. Prevention and Treatment 2003;5. art id 9.
83. Cardemil EV, Reivich KJ, Beevers CG, et al. The prevention of depressive symptoms in low income, minority children: two-year follow-up. Behav Res Ther 2007;45: 313–27.
84. Roberts C, Kane R, Thomson H, et al. The prevention of depressive symptoms in rural school children: a randomized controlled trial. J Consult Clin Psychol 2003; 71:622–8.
85. Stark KD, Hargraves J, Sander J. Treatment of childhood depression: The ACTION treatment program. In: Kendall PC, editor. Child and adolescent therapies: cognitive-behavioral procedures. 3rd edition. New York: Guilford Press; 2006. p. 162–216.
86. De Cuyper S, Timbremont B, Braet C, et al. Treating depressive symptoms in school children: a pilot study. Eur Child Adolesc Psychiatry 2004;13:105–14.
87. Haeffel GJ, Grigorenko EL. Cognitive vulnerability to depression: exploring risk and resilience. Child Adolesc Psychiatr Clin N Am 2007;16:435–48.
88. Downey G, Coyne JC. Children of depressed parents: an integrative review. Psychol Bull 1990;108:50–76.

89. Weissman MM, Wickramaratne P, Nomura Y, et al. Offspring of depressed parents: 20 years later. Arch Gen Psychiatry 2006;163:1001–8.

90. Forbes EE, Shaw DS, Fox NA, et al. Maternal depression, child frontal asymmetry and child affective behavior as factors in child behavior problems. J Child Psychol Psychiatry 2006;47:79–87.

91. Feng X, Shaw DS, Kovacs M, et al. Emotional regulation in preschoolers: the roles of behavioral inhibition, maternal affective behavior and maternal depression. J Child Psychol Psychiatry 2008;49:132–41.

92. Silk JS, Steinberg L, Morris AS. Adolescent's emotion regulation in daily life: links to depressive symptoms and problem behaviors. Child Dev 2003;74:1869–80.

93. Gunlicks M, Weissman MM. Changes in child psychopathology with improvement in parental depression: a systematic review. J Am Acad Child Adolesc Psychiatry 2008;47:379–89.

94. Beardslee WR, Salt P, Versage EM, et al. Sustained change in parents receiving preventive interventions for families with depression. Am J Psychiatry 1997;154:510–5.

95. Beardslee WR, Gladstone TR, Wright EJ, et al. A family-based approach to the prevention of depressive symptoms in children at risk: evidence of parental and child change. Pediatrics 2003;112:119–31.

96. Beardslee WR, Wright EJ, Gladstone TRG, et al. Long-term effects from a randomized trial of two public health preventive interventions for parental depression. J Fam Psychol 2008;21:702–13.

97. Hinshaw SP. The stigmatization of mental illness in children and parents: developmental issues, family concerns and research needs. J Child Psychol Psychiatry 2005;46:714–34.

98. Keenan K, Wakschlag LS. Are oppositional defiant and conduct disorder symptoms normative behaviors in preschoolers? A comparison of referred and non-referred children. Am J Psychiatry 2004;161:356–8.

99. Wakschlag LS, Leventhal BL, Thomas JM. Disruptive behavior disorders & ADHD in preschool children: characterizing heterotypic continuities for a developmentally-informed nosology for DSM V. In: Regier D, First M, Narrow W, editors. Age and gender considerations in psychiatric diagnosis: a research agenda for DSM-V. Washington, DC: American Psychiatric Publishing Inc; 2007.

100. Breitenstein SM, Hill C, Gross D. Understanding disruptive behavior problems in preschool children. J Pediatr Nurs 2009;24:3–12.

101. Reno SM, MCgrath PJ. Predictors of parent training efficacy for child externalizing behavior problems. J Child Psychol Psychiatry 2006;47:99–111.

102. Scott S, Dadds MR. Practitioner review: when parent training doesn't work: theory-driven clinical strategies. J Child Psychol Psychiatry 2009;50:1141–50.

103. Bradshaw CP, Koth CW, Thornton LA, et al. Altering school climate through school-wide positive interventions and supports: findings from a group-randomized effectiveness trial. Prev Sci 2009;10:100–15.

104. Slough NN, McMahon RJ, Bierman KL, et al. Preventing serious conduct problems in school-age youth: The Fast Track Program. Cogn Behav Pract 2008;15:3–17.

105. Greenberg MT, Kusché CA, Cook ET, et al. Promoting emotional competence in school-aged children: the effects of the PATHS curriculum. Development and Psychopathology 1995;7:117–36.

106. The Conduct Problems Prevention Research Group. Initial impact of the fast track prevention trial for conduct problems: I. The high risk sample. J Consult Clin Psychol 1999;67:630–47.

107. Conduct Problems Prevention Research Group. Fast track randomized controlled trial to prevent externalizing psychiatric disorders: Findings from grades 3 to 9. J Am Acad Child Adolesc Psychiatry 2007;46:1250–62.
108. Riggs NR, Greenberg MT, Kusche CA. The mediational role of neurocognition in the behavioral outcomes of a social-emotional prevention program in elementary school students: Effects of the PATHS curriculum. Prev Sci 2006;7:91–102.
109. Greenberg MT. Promoting resilience in children and youth: Preventive interventions and their interface with neuroscience. Ann N Y Acad Sci 2006; 1094:139–50.
110. Izard CE, King KA, Trentacosta CJ. Accelerating the development of emotion competence in head start children: effects on adaptive and maladaptive behavior. Dev Psychopathol 2008;20:369–97.

Medical and Psychiatric Comorbidities in Children and Adolescents: A Guide to Issues and Treatment Approaches

Peggy El-Mallakh, PhD, RN[a],*, Patricia B. Howard, PhD, RN, CNAA, FAAN[a],
Stacey M. Inman, BSBA, JD, BSN, RN[b]

KEYWORDS

- Children • Adolescents
- Comorbid medical and psychiatric illnesses

Chronic medical illnesses among children and adolescents have increased in prevalence since the 1980s; current research estimates that almost 14% of children have a diagnosis of 1 chronic illness, and almost 9% have 2 or more chronic illnesses.[1] Furthermore, much research suggests that mental, emotional, and behavioral problems are common among children and adolescents with chronic medical illnesses.[2,3] To provide competent and holistic care for pediatric populations, nurses need to know the most common psychiatric comorbidities among children and adolescents with chronic medical illnesses. In addition, skill in use of the nursing process is critically important to promote optimal physical and mental health in this population. The purposes of this article are to describe theories of psychological and emotional adjustment to chronic medical illnesses among children and youth, discuss common psychiatric comorbidities, family issues, and current treatment approaches, and identify implications for nurses who care for pediatric populations.

THEORETIC CONSIDERATIONS

Many theoretic models have been developed to identify the factors that contribute to the occurrence of psychological problems in children and adolescents with chronic

---

The authors have no financial disclosures or conflict of interests to report.
[a] University of Kentucky College of Nursing, 202 College of Nursing Building, 760 Rose Street, Lexington, KY 40536-0232, USA
[b] University of Louisville School of Nursing, 555 South Floyd Street, Suite 3019, Louisville, KY 40292, USA
* Corresponding author.
E-mail address: peggy.el-mallakh@uky.edu

Nurs Clin N Am 45 (2010) 541–554
doi:10.1016/j.cnur.2010.06.009
0029-6465/10/$ – see front matter © 2010 Elsevier Inc. All rights reserved.

nursing.theclinics.com

medical conditions. Several theories emphasize the importance of psychological adjustment in determining the effects of living with a chronic medical illness.[2,4] Drotar[4] proposes that the psychological effects of a pediatric chronic illness are multifaceted, and relate to individual and family-centered domains. The ill child's adjustment is associated with self-perceptions of physical appearance, social acceptance,[2] psychological distress, and the presence of a mental illness in the child.[4] High levels of stress are also associated with poor psychological adjustment to chronic illness.[5] In addition, positive psychological adjustment of family members and the ability of family members to offer support are essential in helping the child adjust to the illness.[2,4] Family and child adjustment to a chronic medical illness influences a child's functioning in several areas of life. These include the health care context, specifically illness management, adherence to care, and the child's response to medical procedures, school context, such as academic performance and school attendance, and peer context, such as relationships and interactions with peers.[4] Poor psychological adjustment to a medical illness is characterized by emotional distress, developmental delays, poor adherence to medical treatment, poor peer relationships, poor school performance, and behavioral problems.[4,6]

In addition to models of psychological adjustment, stress and coping models have been developed to illustrate the factors that influence a child's response to a chronic medical illness. In a stress and coping model, the chronic illness is viewed as an extremely demanding stressor that influences several aspects of quality of life, including general well-being and physical, psychological, and social functioning.[7] The stress of a chronic medical illness is offset by the coping resources of the child and their social network; these resources include personal resiliency, coping skills, knowledge about the illness, self-esteem, health beliefs and attitudes, social support, family functioning, and self-care responsibilities associated with the illness. Charron-Prochownik[7] further emphasizes that coping resources serve to buffer the negative effects of a chronic illness, and perceptions of the stress associated with the chronic illness and self-care challenges mediate the negative effect of the illness on quality of life.

Qualitative research has further clarified several broad domains of the experience of living with and adjusting to a chronic medical illness during adolescence.[8] Peer acceptance, development of autonomy, and future prospects are significant issues.[9] Teens value normalcy and are concerned with getting on with life in the context of a chronic medical illness. In addition, families may have a positive influence on teens with chronic medical illnesses when they assist with illness management and guide the teen through treatment. In contrast, families can negatively affect teen's attitudes toward a chronic illness by being overprotective, controlling, and discouraging the teen's independence.[8]

OVERVIEW OF COMORBIDITIES AMONG CHILDREN AND ADOLESCENTS

Research related to psychiatric illnesses in pediatric populations has primarily focused on children and adolescents with asthma, diabetes, cancer, and human immunodeficiency virus (HIV). Family considerations in children and adolescents with comorbidities have also been investigated, particularly related to emotional responses to providing care to a child with a chronic illness. An overview of this research is presented in this section.

Asthma

Asthma is a chronic lung disease characterized by inflammation, airway obstruction, dyspnea, and bronchial hypersensitivity to stimuli.[10,11] It is the most common medical condition among children aged 0 to 17 years. In 2005, approximately 6.5 million children had a diagnosis of asthma, representing almost 9% of all children in the United States.[12] Extensive research on the effects of childhood asthma indicates that it is associated with missed school, high rates of visits to health care providers, frequent hospitalizations, costly medical treatment, and family caregiving burden.[5,12]

Psychological disorders are more common among children and adolescents diagnosed with asthma compared with the general population,[13,14] particularly depressive and anxiety disorders.[15] Common anxiety disorders in pediatric patients include agoraphobia, separation disorder, simple phobias, and panic disorders.[5,16] In 1 study, Richardson and colleagues[17] found that among 767 youth aged 11 to 17 years who were diagnosed with asthma, almost 9% met the diagnostic criteria for an anxiety disorder, 2.5% for a depressive disorder, and almost 5% for comorbid depressive and anxiety disorders. Several risk factors for the development of comorbid anxiety disorders have been identified among children with asthma; these include female gender, having a parent with a high school education or less, being raised in a single parent family, low socioeconomic status, being a recipient of Medicaid-financed health care, recent diagnosis of asthma, and reporting greater functional impairment as a result of asthma.[14,15] Smoking increases the risk for psychiatric comorbidities among youth with asthma[18]; 1 study of 769 participants with asthma who were aged 11 to 17 years indicated that rates of depression were almost 21%, compared with 6.7% of participants who did not smoke. Similarly, rates of one or more anxiety disorders among participants who smoked were almost 30% compared with 12.2% among participants who did not smoke.

Several health-related outcomes are worse among youth with asthma and a comorbid psychiatric disorder compared with those with asthma and no psychiatric comorbidity. Richardson and colleagues,[19] in a study of 767 youth with asthma, found that participants with depression or anxiety reported more asthma-symptom days in a 2-week period compared with those without comorbid depression or anxiety. Furthermore, participants with greater symptoms of depression or anxiety were more likely to report higher levels of asthma symptoms. Health care use and health care costs are significantly higher among youth with asthma and a depressive disorder, with or without an anxiety disorder, compared with youth with asthma and an anxiety disorder alone. Other researchers make the important observation that depression and anxiety in youth with asthma contribute to negative outcomes in non–asthma-related domains, such as low quality of life and impaired physical functioning.[14]

Diabetes

The Centers for Disease Control and Prevention (CDC)[20] states that approximately 186,300, or 0.2%, of people less than 20 years of age in the United States have been diagnosed with diabetes. It is unknown how many youth in this age group have diabetes and remain undiagnosed. The annual rate of new diagnosis from 2002 to 2003 was 19.0 per 100,000 for type 1 diabetes (T1DM). In contrast, rates of type 2 diabetes (T2DM) were 5.3 per 100,000. Although T2DM was rare in youth, there was a slightly higher incidence rate in youth aged 10 to 19 years, as opposed to children less than 10 years old. T2DM also occurs more frequently in minority youth than in non-Hispanic white populations. In fact, among Asian/Pacific Islander and American Indian youth aged 10 to 19 years, the rate of new cases of T2DM was greater than the rate for T1DM. Further, African American and Hispanic youth aged 10 to 19 years had similar incidence rates for both T1DM and T2DM. The highest youth incidence of

T1DM was among the non-Hispanic white population. Statistics from 1999 to 2000 indicated that among US adolescents aged 12 to 19 years, 7.0% were diagnosed with impaired fasting glucose, also known as prediabetes.[20]

Children and adolescents with diabetes are likely to feel burdened by diabetes management, and as a result, depressive symptoms may develop. Studies have shown that children and adolescents with T1DM experience depression at a rate up to 3 times the rate of depression in the general population of the same age group. Depression may then affect the child's diabetes outcomes.[21] Indeed, a research study of 231 adolescent outpatients with T1DM indicated that those with high levels of depressive symptoms were at increased risk for hospitalization for diabetes and associated physical complications.[22] These findings underscore the potential for high-risk behaviors in this population. For example, a psychiatric disorder associated with poor diabetes outcomes is intentional self-harm, which may be manifested by overdoses of insulin. In addition, eating disorders and associated intentional insulin omission are increasing in incidence among adolescents with T1DM.[23]

Childhood diabetes has an effect on the child, the parents, and even the dynamics of the family. Indeed, the presence of a child with diabetes in the family can negatively influence the effective functioning of the entire family. Family conflict is associated with poor adherence to the diabetic regimen and poor control of the diabetes. In this way a vicious cycle is perpetuated whereby the child's resistance to diabetes management leads to family conflict, which in turn leads to poor diabetes outcomes and consequent increase in family conflict.[21] These findings reinforce the importance of family responsibility for the child's daily treatment while assuming all other family responsibilities, as well as the importance of adaptive parental coping. Research has indicated that there are differences in how mothers and fathers cope with such stress. Mothers used more planning and problem solving, whereas fathers tended to use distancing to cope.[24] Chisholm and colleagues[25] found that better maternal diabetes knowledge correlated with better outcomes for the child, including fewer relationship difficulties.

Cancer

Between 2004 and 2006, the most common cancers diagnosed among people less than 20 years of age were leukemia (45.3%), with lymphoma leukemia the most frequently diagnosed at 34.4%; lymphomas, with Hodgkin lymphoma the most frequently diagnosed at 23.6%; and brain/central nervous system (CNS) tumors (28.3%), with astrocytomas the most frequently diagnosed at 14.6%.[26] A diagnosis of cancer is life threatening, and the experience of aggressive cancer treatment during childhood and adolescence has a significant effect on several aspects of growth and developmental issues and emotional/behavioral outcomes.[27,28] Jones[28] reports that lengthy hospitalizations, frequent supervision, and isolation from peers prevent adolescents from achieving critical developmental milestones, such as peer relationships, social identity formation, and cognitive maturity. Psychological distress is a common response to invasive painful procedures, chemotherapy, and prolonged hospitalizations. Some research indicates that distress tends to be most intense during the early phases of treatment, with decreased intensity occurring over the course of illness.[29] In addition, the source of distress related to the cancer experience depends on the child's age.[30] Children aged 0 to 3 years are most distressed by confinement (being held during procedures, having to keep still during treatment, and being isolated because of immunosuppression), pain, and worry about medical procedures. For children aged 4 to 7 years, a feeling of alienation from peers causes the most distress; among children aged 8 to 12 years, worry about death is the most significant source of distress. In addition, adolescents aged 13 to 19 years cite changes in appearance as a result of a diagnosis of cancer and treatment as the most significant source of distress.[30]

Research related to depression in children and adolescents has yielded varying results in the pediatric population. In a study by Hockenberry and colleagues,[31] treatment with cisplastin, doxorubicin, or ifosfamide was associated with increased fatigue and sleep disturbances, and higher levels of fatigue were associated with higher levels of depression. In addition, children and adolescents with higher levels of fatigue reported more emotional and behavioral problems. However, Dejong and Fombonne[32] reviewed several studies on depression in pediatric patients with cancer, and found that low prevalence rates of depression were reported in most studies. However, they attribute the findings to methodological challenges in measuring depression in medically ill children, particularly related to the issue of whether a depression instrument tested in a healthy pediatric population is a valid measure of depression in a pediatric patient who has cancer. These researchers propose that children diagnosed with cancer may be resilient and able to tolerate the stress of cancer treatment if they receive emotional support from parents. This suggestion underscores the importance of assessing parental response to pediatric cancer, the presence of psychological distress or depression in parents, and the need for health care workers to encourage and support parental efforts that promote adaptive coping in children with cancer.

As a result of the development of effective chemotherapy, up to 78% of childhood patients with cancer survive into adulthood.[28] Thus, cancer researchers have the opportunity to investigate the long-term consequences of childhood cancer treatment on multiple aspects of emotional, cognitive, and psychosocial characteristics in adult survivors of childhood cancer. In 1 study, young adult survivors reported symptoms of posttraumatic stress disorder related to childhood cancer treatment; the researchers suggest that this can cause survivors to avoid seeking medical treatment.[33,34] Zebrack and colleagues,[35] in a study of 5736 long-term survivors of childhood leukemia, Hodgkin disease, and non-Hodgkin lymphoma, findings suggested that study participants had an increased risk of reporting depression compared with their healthy siblings, and that intensive treatment with chemotherapy added to the risk of depression and somatic distress.

Several research reports identify adverse outcomes resulting from cancer treatment. These outcomes include functional limitations, short stature, obesity, infertility, and developmental delays, which can increase the risk for psychological distress among adults who survived childhood cancer. In addition, treatment of brain and CNS tumors often results in hearing loss, cerebrovascular incidents, and paralysis in those treated for childhood CNS cancer treatments.[36] Neurocognitive functioning is often compromised among adults who were treated for brain and CNS tumors during childhood.[36] Treatment with high-dose cranial irradiation is associated with neuroanatomical changes, such as cortical atrophy, vascular damage, and destruction of white matter.[32] Negative psychosocial outcomes resulting from treatment with cranial irradiation include poor school performance, lower IQ, and reduced likelihood of college attendance among survivors of childhood cancer. In a study of 802 adult survivors of childhood CNS malignancies, participants who received cranial irradiation or had a ventriculoperitoneal shunt placement demonstrated significant levels of cognitive impairments, particularly in the areas of speed of task performance, information processing speed, multitasking, and long-term and working memory. These neurocognitive impairments were significantly associated with lower educational attainment, lower household income, less full-time employment, and fewer marriages, all of which increase the risk for development of stress, maladaptive coping, and psychiatric disorders in adulthood.[36]

Although most survivors of childhood cancer are emotionally healthy, a significant subset has reported problems with poor psychological health and mental health–related quality of life.[37] Glover and colleagues[38] investigated psychiatric outcomes among 555 young adult survivors of acute lymphocytic leukemia (ALL); findings indicated that 24% of participants reported mood disturbances, as measured by the Profiles of Mood States (POMS). Age at diagnosis, gender, educational status, and type of treatment for ALL significantly increased the risk of developing mood disturbances in the study sample. For example, those who were diagnosed before the age of 12.5 years were 3.7 times more likely to report mood disturbances. Although males in the study sample were almost 4 times more likely to report mood disturbances, female participants who required special education were 6 times more likely to report mood disturbances. In addition, high school dropouts who had required special education were 48 times more likely to report mood disturbances, and participants who received high doses of methotrexate and cranial irradiation were 1.7 times more likely to report mood disturbances.

HIV and AIDS

The Centers for Disease Control[39] estimates that between 1992 and 2007, more than 9029 children less than 13 years old, 1169 children between the ages of 13 and 14 years, and 6089 adolescents had a diagnosis of AIDS. HIV and AIDS cause several serious complications in the pediatric population, both in the CNS and in other organ systems. Neurocognitive impairments in children are related to HIV encephalopathy,[40] impaired brain growth, progressive motor dysfunction, and failure to reach developmental milestones.[41] In addition, Rao and colleagues[41] stress that HIV infection in children causes growth stunting, chronic dermatologic conditions, lipodystrophy, and lipoatrophy, which can negatively affect self-esteem and body image.

Several comorbid psychiatric diagnoses have been identified in children and adolescents with HIV/AIDS.[42,43] Mellins and colleagues[42] used the Child Behavioral Checklist and the Diagnostic Interview Schedule for Children (DISC) to identify psychiatric comorbidities in 47 youth, aged 9 to 16 years, with perinatally acquired AIDS. Findings suggest that most participants had been informed about their AIDS diagnosis, and that more than half (55%) had a comorbid psychiatric disorder. The most prevalent diagnoses were anxiety disorders (40%), which included social phobia, separation anxiety, agoraphobia, panic disorder, and obsessive compulsive disorders. In addition, 23% had a behavioral disorder, including attention-deficit hyperactivity disorder, conduct disorder, or oppositional-defiant disorder. Gaughan and colleagues[43] report that psychiatric hospitalizations among children and adolescents with HIV infection are more frequent compared with children who are not infected. In a study of 1808 children and youth with HIV, the most frequent reasons for hospitalization were depression and behavioral disorders. Other researchers have observed tantrums, conduct and behavioral problems, labile emotions, and social withdrawal among children and adolescents with HIV.[44]

In general, youth with HIV experience multiple psychosocial stressors that increase their risk for developing psychiatric comorbidities.[45] These include the stigma and discrimination resulting from a diagnosis of HIV/AIDS, emotional distress because of having a potentially fatal illness, and the need to make a commitment to lifelong adherence to a complex and demanding medication regimen to avoid a fatal outcome. However, some distinct differences have been identified in the psychological issues of youth with perinatally acquired HIV and youth who contracted HIV as preteens or adolescents. Youth with perinatally acquired HIV have HIV-infected parents, and must cope with parental behaviors that led to the parental diagnosis of HIV/AIDS, particularly substance abuse. In addition, many youth with perinatally acquired HIV are AIDS orphans, and must cope with the trauma and grief associated with parental loss, being placed in foster care and consequent vulnerability to early deprivation, abuse or neglect, or separation from siblings.[45] In contrast, youth who contract HIV during their preteen or adolescent years often have behavioral, emotional, and social issues that placed them at risk for contracting HIV; these include truancy and runaway behaviors, multiple losses of supportive relationships, engagement in the juvenile justice system or incarceration, disruption of parent/teen relationships, parental abandonment or neglect, and substance abuse, particularly alcohol and marijuana.[46,47] Sexual abuse and assault are common among youth who contract HIV during their preteen or adolescent years. In a study of 50 HIV-positive youth, Davey and colleagues[46] found that 89% had histories of sexual assault, and that 11% had contracted HIV as a result of sexual assault. In addition, parental support among teens who contracted HIV as a result of behavioral problems was poor both before and after they contracted HIV. Clearly, youth who contract HIV during adolescence often struggle with the issue of how to disclose their HIV status to their parents, and therefore need support from health care providers during the process of disclosure. Davey and colleagues[46] reported that in their study, teens who had difficult relationships with their parents or poor family support were at times kicked out of the home after disclosing their HIV status.

Recent advances in antiretroviral treatment (ART) have changed the course and prognosis of HIV.[45] Whereas HIV was a fatal illness before the development of ART, it is now considered a chronic, long-term illness that can be successfully managed for an extended length of time.[41] AS a result of these advances in ART, Rao and colleagues[41] stress that the life expectancy of children and adolescents with HIV/AIDS is increasing; thus effective treatment is needed to reduce HIV encephalopathy and associated neurocognitive impairments, maintain normal growth and development into adulthood, and improve emotional well-being and quality of life. Treatment with highly active antiretroviral therapy (HAART) and other medications that penetrate the blood-brain barrier can dramatically reduce the incidence of HIV encephalopathy.[40] However, few psychosocial interventions exist to address issues of emotional well-being, developmental issues, and quality of life in this population. In particular, several researchers have stressed the need for interventions to address issues related to long-term planning for education and employment, relationship issues, sexuality, and childbearing among HIV-positive youth who are approaching adulthood.[48]

Family Considerations

Families are integral to the health and well-being of children.[49] For this reason, pediatricians increasingly encourage a family-centered approach to pediatric care; optimal attention to the family in pediatric care can allow practitioners to identify families and children at risk for poor outcomes in response to chronic childhood illness. In general, parenting a chronically medically ill child is physically and emotionally exhausting, highly stressful, and a source of constant worry.[50] Furthermore, a comorbid psychiatric diagnosis in a child with a chronic medical illness can profoundly influence parental perception of caregiver role strain. Chavira and colleagues[13] have observed that caregiver role strain was significantly higher among parents of children with comorbid chronic medical illnesses and anxiety disorders compared with caregiver role strain for children with a sole diagnosis of an anxiety disorder or for children with a single diagnosis of a chronic medical disorder. In addition, Morowska and colleagues[51] report that emotional and resistive child behaviors surrounding asthma illness management, such as anxiety, opposition, and aggression, are associated with more problems in the caregiving role and lower parental confidence in engaging in asthma management tasks.

CURRENT TREATMENT APPROACHES

Care of the children and youth with chronic medical illnesses and psychiatric comorbidities requires a multifaceted approach that encompasses physical symptoms, psychosocial concerns, and family considerations. A multidisciplinary team of pediatric and child/adolescent psychiatric clinicians is ideally suited to address the extensive needs of this population. Assessment of the child with a chronic medical illness should always include common psychiatric illnesses, particularly depression, anxiety, and posttraumatic stress disorder. Suicidal ideation, attempts, and previous history of suicide must be assessed, particularly among those who are diagnosed with depression.[43] Child and parental reports of symptoms should be included in the assessment. The Kiddie-Schedule of Affective Disorders and Schizophrenia (K-SADS), the DISC, and the Child Behavior Checklist have been used in research and clinical practice with this population. However, as indicated previously, these tools have been developed and used primarily in pediatric populations without chronic medical illnesses, and should be used cautiously in a pediatric population with comorbidities. The use of these tools in pediatric patients with comorbidities may underrate the full range of psychiatric symptoms that accompany a chronic medical illness in a pediatric population, and thus provide an inaccurate picture of psychiatric illnesses among those with comorbidities.

Some research studies have been conducted to investigate the effectiveness of interventions for children and adolescents with medical and psychiatric comorbidities. However, these studies have methodological issues, such as small sample sizes and modest effect sizes, that limit generalizability to varying age groups and types of physical illnesses within this population.[4,52] Continued research on the effectiveness of these interventions is warranted to expand the evidence base for pediatric and psychiatric nurses in their efforts to promote optimal outcomes in this population; however, several guidelines for nursing care are available.

Interventions for Children

Nursing interventions for children should be age and developmentally appropriate. Chesson and colleagues[53] acknowledge the limitations of talk therapy and further state that play and drawing are "natural modes of communication for children, especially before pre-adolescence".(p 333) Play therapy should ideally involve the parents through participation in art therapy, puppet play, reading activities, and therapeutic medical play with their children.[54] Studies using cognitive behavioral therapy, psychosocial support, and social skills training have been conducted among children with cancer and their families; these studies have emphasized education, support, problem solving, family functioning, assertiveness training, and positive school reintegration. Findings from these studies suggest that these interventions can reduce behavioral problems and improve quality of life, constructive problem solving, social support, and family functioning.[55–58] Among children with asthma, self-management training combined with relaxation-breathing exercises can reduce anxiety.[59] In addition, computerized education/self-management programs have been shown to improve adherence to self-care.[5]

Several illness management strategies have been recommended to reduce emotional distress and enhance the perception of control over an illness among children and adolescents with comorbidities. For example, Brown and colleagues[5] maintain that self-regulatory skills training aims to "convince children that they are able to effectively manage their illness"[(p.60)]. A wide variety of strategies are used in self-regulatory skills training, such as medication management, inter- and intrapersonal skill development, and relapse prevention. Similarly, self-management skills training emphasizes a child's or adolescent's central role in the management of their illness; strategies include enhancement of illness management skills, maintenance of life roles, goal setting, confidence building, and decision making.[5]

Interventions for Adolescents

From a developmental perspective, adolescents are concerned with independence, identity formation, and peer relationships.[48] Thus, interventions for adolescents with comorbidities should ideally create an environment to interact with peers and provide an outlet for exploring how the experience of a chronic medical illness defines who they are as a person. Peer support groups are increasingly used among adolescents with chronic illnesses to promote treatment adherence and provide a forum for exploring and discussing health beliefs, spirituality, family issues and conflicts, and concerns about illness relapses.[5,60] A family-centered support group has been used among adolescents with perinatally acquired HIV to deal with the issues and challenges they face; these include dating, sexual experimentation, disclosure of HIV status to friends, and planning for the future.[48] The group further provides an outlet for expressing existential distress associated with a diagnosis of HIV (why me?) and feelings of abandonment following the death of a parent from HIV.

Technologically savvy children and adolescents can use digital technology to express emotions that occur in response to isolation, loss of control, and anxiety associated with hospitalizations and intensive treatment for cancer. For example, therapeutic songwriting, music video production, and digital video production interventions have been shown to decrease anxiety in pediatric patients undergoing bone marrow transplants.[61] In addition, electronic support groups, such as STARBRIGHT World, are available to hospitalized pediatric patients and allow them to interact with other hospitalized pediatric patients in an online community.[5] Participation in STARBRIGHT World has been shown to reduce pain intensity, pain aversiveness, and anxiety in hospitalized youth aged 9 to 19 years.[62]

Adolescents with chronic medical illnesses are in need of counseling for illness risk reduction and health promotion behaviors. Teens with asthma should be educated on the risks of smoking and the effects of smoking on anxiety symptoms.[18] Jones[28] points out that the long-term consequences of cancer treatment, such as delayed sexual development, obesity, and short stature, may lower self-esteem and increase a sense of social isolation and alienation from peers; these emotional responses can, in turn, increase the risk of substance abuse. Thus, nurses need to assess risk for substance abuse and provide risk reduction counseling among adolescent survivors of cancer.

Prevention efforts are also critically important among teens who are at risk for contracting chronic medical illnesses. For example, teens must be assessed for risky behaviors and social factors that make them vulnerable to contracting HIV, such as substance use, particularly alcohol and marijuana, high-risk sexual activity, history of sexual abuse, younger age at sexual debut, dropping out of school, associating with peers who engage in high-risk behaviors, and contentious relationships with parents or guardians.[47,63] Bachanas and colleagues[63] recommend a primary care–based multidisciplinary approach designed specifically for adolescents that involves mental health practitioners in the provision of prevention-based interventions for high-risk behaviors.

Interventions for Families

Drotar[4] stresses that interventions are needed to reduce the emotional distress among family members of children with chronic illnesses. Families, particularly parents, need considerable support in the care of children and youth with comorbidities.[64] Parents are in most need of support immediately following the child's diagnosis; Coffey[50] reports that parents may experience shock, helplessness, depression, suicidal ideation, a sense of isolation, and fear immediately following their child's diagnosis. In addition, the first year following diagnosis is an equally distressing time for family members; this time period is typically characterized by learning to implement complex treatment regimens in the care of the child, adjusting to the demands of caregiving along with having to attend to all other family needs, emotional exhaustion, hypervigilance, worry about the urgency of symptoms, and indecision about when to notify the health care provider about changes in symptoms.[50,65,66] Critical milestones in the child's life are also difficult for parents, particularly during the adolescent years, when parents are faced with transferring primary responsibility for illness management to the child.[50] In addition, parental caregivers of adolescents with chronic medical illnesses need support in coping with a range of factors that contribute to caregiver role strain, such as resistance to taking medications, Ledlie[48] further observes that health care providers need to assess concerns of parental caregivers of youth with perinatally acquired HIV, particularly guilt about causing the HIV infection in the youth and decision making regarding the appropriate time for disclosing the diagnosis to the HIV-positive youth.

Several strategies tailored to the needs of parents have been identified.[64,66] Nurses are encouraged to help parents normalize the caregiving role by acknowledging the challenges that parents face in providing care for their ill children. The development of collaborative partnerships between parents and nurses is crucial, and can be fostered by acknowledging parental expertise and soliciting their observations and suggestions. In addition, nurses need to explore parents' emotional well-being and personal needs and encourage parents to participate in parental peer support groups.[66] Indeed, parents have reported that peer support groups are invaluable in helping them cope with providing care to a chronically ill child, stating that only another parent of a child with a chronic illness can fully understand the intense emotional distress that characterizes the experience.[67]

SUMMARY

Chronic medical illness among children and adolescents is a growing concern with implications for informal and formal caregivers. When coupled with a psychiatric comorbidity, implications grow exponentially. Nurses who care for child and adolescent populations play a crucial role in optimizing physical and mental health when they interface with patients and their caregivers. Evidence-based interventions can promote positive outcomes and enhance quality of life, whereas failure to use evidence-based approaches has serious consequences to the health of youth with medical and psychiatric comorbidities.

REFERENCES

1. National survey of children's health, 2007. Available at: http://www.nschdata.org. Accessed February 13, 2010.

2. Immelt S. Psychological adjustment in young children with chronic medical conditions. J Pediatr Nurs 2006;21(5):362–77.
3. Hysing M, Elgen I, Gillberg C, et al. Chronic physical illness and mental health in children. Results from a large-scale population study. J Child Psychol Psychiatry 2007;48(8):785–92.
4. Drotar D. Psychological interventions in childhood chronic illness. Washington, DC: American Psychological Association Press; 2006.
5. Brown RT, Daly BP, Rickel AU. Chronic illness in children and adolescents. Cambridge (MA): Hogrefe & Huber; 2007.
6. Harris ES, Canning RD, Kelleher KJ. A comparison of measures of adjustment, symptoms, impairment among children with chronic medical conditions. J Am Acad Child Adolesc Psychiatry 1996;35(8):1025–32.
7. Charron-Prochownik D. Special needs of the chronically ill child during middle childhood: application of a stress-coping paradigm. J Pediatr Nurs 2002;17(6):407–13.
8. Taylor RM, Gibson F, Franck LS. The experience of living with a chronic illness during adolescence: a critical review of the literature. J Clin Nurs 2008;17:3083–91.
9. McEwan MJ, Espie CA, Metcalfe J, et al. Quality of life and psychosocial development in adolescents with epilepsy: a qualitative investigation using focus group methods. Seizure 2004;13:15–31.
10. Hampel P, Rudolph H, Stachow R, et al. Multimodal patient education program with stress management for childhood and adolescent asthma. Patient Educ Couns 2003;49:59–66.
11. Brashers VI. Alterations in pulmonary function. In: McCance KL, Heuther SE, editors. Pathophysiology: the biologic basis for disease in adults and children. 5th edition. St Louis (MO): Elsevier Mosby; 2006. p. 1205–48.
12. Akinbami LJ. The state of childhood asthma, United States, 1980–2005. Advance data from vital and health statistics, 381. Washington, DC: Centers for Disease Control, National Center for Health Statistics, US Dept of Health and Human Services; 2006.
13. Chavira DA, Garland AF, Daley S, et al. The impact of medical comorbidity on mental health and functional health outcomes among children with anxiety disorders. J Dev Behav Pediatr 2008;29(5):394–402.
14. Katon W, Lozano P, Russo J, et al. The prevalence of DSM-IV anxiety and depressive disorders in youth with asthma compared to controls. J Adolesc Health 2007; 41(5):455–63.
15. Katon WJ, Richardson L, Lozano P, et al. The relationship of asthma and anxiety disorders. Psychosom Med 2004;66:349–55.
16. Ortega AN, Huertas SE, Canino G, et al. Childhood asthma, chronic illness, and psychiatric disorders. J Nerv Ment Dis 2002;190(5):275–81.
17. Richardson LP, Russo JE, Lozano P, et al. The effect of comorbid anxiety and depressive disorders on health care utilization and costs among adolescents with asthma. Gen Hosp Psychiatry 2008;30:398–406.
18. Bush T, Richardson L, Katon W, et al. Anxiety and depressive disorders are associated with smoking in adolescents with asthma. J Adolesc Health 2007;40:425–32.
19. Richardson LP, Lozano P, Russo J, et al. Asthma symptom burden: relationship to asthma severity and anxiety and depression symptoms. Pediatrics 2006;118(5): 1042–51.
20. Centers for Disease Control and Prevention. National diabetes fact sheet: general information and national estimates on diabetes in the United States, 2007. Atlanta (GA): US Department of Health; 2008.

21. Williams LB, Laffelt LM, Hood KK. Diabetes-specific family conflict and psychological distress in paediatric type 1 diabetes. Diabet Med 2009;26(9):908–14.
22. Stewart SM, Rao U, Emslie GJ, et al. Depressive symptoms predict hospitalization for adolescents with type 1 diabetes mellitus. Pediatrics 2005;115(5):1315–9.
23. Garrison MM, Katon WJ, Richardson LP. The impact of psychiatric comorbidities on readmissions for diabetes in youth. Diabetes Care 2005;28(9):2150–4.
24. Azar R, Solomon CR. Coping strategies of parents facing child diabetes mellitus. J Pediatr Nurs 2001;16(6):418–28.
25. Chisholm V, Atkinson L, Donaldson C, et al. Predictors of treatment adherence in young children with type 1 diabetes. J Adv Nurs 2007;57(5):482–93.
26. National Cancer Institute. Surveillance epidemiology end result (SEER) cancer statistics review, 1975–2006. Available at: http://seer.cancer.gov/csr/1975_2006/index.html. Accessed February 18, 2010.
27. Barrera M, Atenafu E, Pinto J. Behavioral, social and educational outcomes after pediatric stem cell transplantation and related factors. Cancer 2009;115:880–9.
28. Jones BL. Promoting healthy development among survivors of adolescent cancer. Fam Community Health 2008;31(15 Suppl 1):S61–70.
29. Sawyer M, Antoniou G, Toogood I, et al. Childhood cancer: a 4-year prospective study of the psychological adjustment of children and parents. J Pediatr Hematol Oncol 2000;22(3):214–20.
30. Hedström M, Haglund K, Skolin I, et al. Distressing events for children and adolescents with cancer: child, parent and nurse perceptions. J Pediatr Oncol Nurs 2003;20(3):120–32.
31. Hockenberry MJ, Hooke MC, Gregurich M, et al. Symptom clusters in children and adolescents receiving cisplatin, doxorubicin, or ifosfamide. Oncol Nurs Forum 2010;37(1):E16–27.
32. Dejong M, Fombonne E. Depression in paediatric cancer: an overview. Psychooncology 2006;15:553–66.
33. Hobbie WL, Stuber M, Meeske K, et al. Symptoms of posttraumatic stress in young adult survivors of childhood cancer. J Clin Oncol 2000;18(24):4060–6.
34. Rourke MT, Hobbie WL, Schwartz L, et al. Posttraumatic stress disorder (PTSD) in young adult survivors of childhood cancer. Pediatr Blood Cancer 2007;49:117–82.
35. Zebrack BJ, Zeltzer LK, Whitton J, et al. Psychological outcomes in long-term survivors of childhood leukemia, Hodgkin's disease, and non-Hodgkin's lymphoma: a report from the Childhood Cancer Survivor Study. Pediatrics 2002;110(1):42–52.
36. Ellenberg L, Liu Q, Gioia G, et al. Neurocognitive status in long-term survivors of childhood CNS malignancies: a report from the Childhood Cancer Survivor Study. Neuropsychology 2009;23(6):705–17.
37. Zeltzer LK, Recklitis C, Buchbinder D, et al. Psychological status in childhood cancer survivors: a report from the Childhood Cancer Survivor Study. J Clin Oncol 2009;27(14):2396–404.
38. Glover DA, Byrne J, Mills JL, et al. Impact of CNS treatment on mood in adult survivors of childhood leukemia: a report from the Children's Cancer Group. J Clin Oncol 2003;21(23):4395–401.
39. Centers for Disease Control and Prevention, Department of Health and Human Services. HIV/AIDS surveillance report: cases of HIV infection and AIDS in the United States and dependent areas. Available at: http://www.cdc.gov/hiv/topics/surveillance/basic.htm. Accessed April 3, 2010.

40. Patel K, Ming X, Williams PL, et al. Impact of HAART and CNS-penetrating anti-retroviral regimens on HIV encephalopathy among perinatally infected children and adolescents. AIDS 2009;23(14):1893.
41. Rao R, Sagar R, Kabra SK, et al. Psychiatric morbidity in HIV-infected children. AIDS Care 2007;19(6):828–33.
42. Mellins CA, Brackis-Cott E, Dolezal C, et al. Psychiatric disorders in youth with perinatally acquired human immunodeficiency virus infection. Pediatr Infect Dis J 2006;25(5):432–7.
43. Gaughan DM, Hughes MD, Oleske JM, et al. Psychiatric hospitalizations among children and youths with human immunodeficiency virus infection. Pediatrics 2004;113(6):e544–51.
44. Scharko AM. DSM psychiatric disorders in the context of pediatric HIV/AIDS. AIDS Care 2006;18(5):441–5.
45. Domek GJ. Facing adolescence and adulthood: the importance of mental health care in the global pediatric AIDS epidemic. J Dev Behav Pediatr 2009;30(2):147–50.
46. Davey MP, Foster J, Milton K, et al. Collaborative approaches to increasing family support for HIV positive youth. Fam Syst Health 2009;27(1):39–52.
47. Kadivar H, Garvie PA, Sinnock C, et al. Psychosocial profile of HIV-infected adolescents in a southern US urban cohort. AIDS Care 2006;18(6):544–9.
48. Ledlie SW. The psychosocial issues of children with perinatally acquired HIV disease becoming adolescents: a growing challenge for providers. AIDS Patient Care 2001;15(5):231–6.
49. American Academy of Pediatrics. Family pediatrics: report of the task force on the family. Pediatrics 2003;111(6):1541–71.
50. Coffey JS. Parenting a child with a chronic illness: a metasynthesis. Pediatr Nurs 2006;32(1):51–9.
51. Morawska A, Stelzer J, Burgess S. Parenting asthmatic children: identification of parenting challenges. J Asthma 2008;45:465–72.
52. Brewer M, Melnyk BM. Effective coping/mental health interventions for critically ill adolescents: an evidence review. Pediatr Nurs 2007;33(4):361–73.
53. Chesson RA, Chisholm D, Zaw W. Counseling children with chronic physical illness. Patient Educ Couns 2004;55:331–8.
54. Melnyk BM, Small L, Carno MA. The effectiveness of parent-focused interventions in improving coping/mental health outcomes of critically ill children and their parents: an evidence base to guide clinical practice. Pediatr Nurs 2004;30(2):143.
55. Varni JW, Katz ER, Colegrove R, et al. The impact of social skills training on the adjustment of children with newly diagnosed cancer. J Pediatr Psychol 1993;18:751–67.
56. Schwartz CE, Feinberg RG, Jilinskaia E, et al. An evaluation of a psychosocial intervention for survivors of childhood cancer: paradoxical effects of a response shift over time. Psycho-oncology 1999;8:344–54.
57. Kazak AE, Simms S, Barakat L, et al. Surviving Cancer Competently Intervention Program (SCCIP): a cognitive-behavioral and family therapy intervention for adolescent survivors of childhood cancer and their families. Fam Process 1999;38:823–31.
58. Sahler OJ, Fairclough DL, Phipps S, et al. Using problem-solving skills training to reduce negative affectivity in mothers of children with newly diagnosed cancer: report of a multisite randomized trial. J Consult Clin Psychol 2005;73:272–83.
59. Chiang L, Ma W, Huang J, et al. Effect of relaxation-breathing training an anxiety and asthma signs/symptoms of children with moderate-to-severe asthma: a randomized controlled trial. Int J Nurs Stud 2009;46:1061–70.

60. Marovic S, Snyders F. Addressing complexities of medical noncompliance in serious childhood illness: collaborating at the interface of providers, families, and health care systems. Fam Syst Health 2008;26(3):237–49.

61. Robb SL, Ebberts AG. Songwriting and digital video production interventions for pediatric patients undergoing bone marrow transplantation, Part I: an analysis of depression and anxiety levels according to phase of treatment. J Pediatr Oncol Nurs 2003;20(1):2–15.

62. Holden G, Bearison DJ, Rode DC, et al. The effects of a computer network on pediatric pain and anxiety. J Technol Hum Serv 2000;17:27–47.

63. Bachanas PJ, Morris MK, Lewis-Gess JK, et al. Psychological adjustment, substance use, HIV knowledge, and risky sexual behavior in at-risk minority females: developmental differences during adolescence. J Pediatr Psychol 2002;27(4):373–84.

64. Sallfors C, Hallberg L. A parental perspective on living with a chronically ill child: a qualitative study. Fam Syst Health 2003;21(2):193–204.

65. Clements D, Copeland L, Loftus M. Critical times for families with a chronically ill child. Pediatr Nurs 1990;16(2):157–61.

66. Kratz L, Uding N, Trahms CM, et al. Managing childhood chronic illness: parent perspectives and implications for parent-provider relationships. Fam Syst Health 2009;27(4):303–13.

67. Johnson B. Mothers' perceptions of parenting children with disabilities. MCN Am J Matern Child Nurs 2000;25(3):127–32.

Interventions for Anxiety in the Critically Ill: A Guide for Nurses and Families

Jenny L. Sauls, DSN, RN, CNE*, Lita F. Warise, EdD, RN, CNE

KEYWORDS

• Anxiety • Critically ill • Nurses • Families

Anxiety, an inevitable feeling for most patients[1,2] and families[3] during the critical care experience, can be positively impacted by critical care nurses. Painful procedures, artificial ventilation, endotracheal suctioning, difficulty communicating, constant artificial lighting, alarms, discomfort, unfamiliar noises, lack of meaningful stimuli, and fear of the unknown are just a few of the stressors that have been identified in the literature resulting in anxiety for critically ill patients.[4–7] Fear of the death of a loved one, uncertain prognosis, financial concerns, emotional turmoil, disruption of roles and routines, and unfamiliar hospital environment are variables that create anxiety for families.[3] Critical care nurses can help to create an environment that will result in improved outcomes for these patients and their families. The interventions provided by critical care nurses can help to control and/or alleviate the negative consequences that accompany unrelieved anxiety. Included in this article is a description of anxiety, related factors, and specific interventions that can be used by critical care nurses to manage anxiety experienced by patients and families in the critical care environment.

Antai-Onong[8] defines anxiety as an affective or emotional response to a stressor that manifests through biologic, behavioral, motor, and psychological indicators. Biologic indicators might include an increase in respiratory rate, increase in heart rate, an increase in blood pressure, diaphoresis, and shortness of breath. These symptoms are more commonly known as the stress response. Behavioral indicators in critically ill patients might include avoidance, failure to cooperate, agitation, and increased dependence. Motor responses exhibited by patients in a critical care setting include tension, tremors, and restlessness, whereas a sense of doom, intense fear, powerlessness, disorientation, and confusion represent the psychological indicators.

School of Nursing, Middle Tennessee State University, PO Box 81, 1301 East Main Street, Murfreesboro, TN 37132, USA
* Corresponding author.
E-mail address: jsauls@mtsu.edu

Nurs Clin N Am 45 (2010) 555–567
doi:10.1016/j.cnur.2010.06.006
0029-6465/10/$ – see front matter © 2010 Elsevier Inc. All rights reserved.

Although a mild to moderate level of anxiety may be helpful in mounting a defense against a real or perceived threat, an ongoing state of anxiety is detrimental to critically ill patients who are already physically compromised. The ongoing stress response that occurs as a result of the perceived threat triggers a release of chemical mediators, such as epinephrine, norepinephrine, and cortisol, which assist in the fight-or-flight response. These same hormones that provide more energy to fight off the foe also contribute to an increased workload on the heart by increasing the heart rate and blood pressure through vasoconstriction and increased cardiac output in response to an increased need for oxygen. For patients who are already suffering from physical stress, the added emotional stress on the heart and circulatory system complicates the situation by further increasing energy requirements as a result of increased myocardial oxygen consumption. These responses have been shown to be detrimental in several different patient populations with increased risks of morbidity and mortality.[9–14] Because of the potentially serious nature of anxiety in critically ill patients, it is important for critical care nurses to identify indicators of anxiety early to intervene in a timely manner to prevent or reduce overall negative consequences.

Through the use of the nursing process, critical care nurses can accurately assess, plan, and offer a number of interventions that can be effective tools for creating an environment that is safe, healing, and humane. Creating a healthy environment addresses the goal established by the American Association of Critical Care Nurses Healthy Work Environment Campaign, which acknowledges the contributions of the patient, the family, and the nurse and emphasizes communication and collaboration as key factors in achieving the goal.[6]

ASSESSMENT

Accurate assessment is the first step in the process. Research findings indicate that critical care nurses primarily rely on physiologic and behavioral indicators for identifying anxiety in their critically ill patients.[5,15] Even though multiple physiologic, behavioral, cognitive, and motor manifestations for anxiety have been identified, studies indicate that the patient's self-report is the most accurate measure of anxiety.[1,16,17] Research also indicates that nurses' rating of anxiety levels when compared with patients' self-rating of anxiety have little to no relationship.[16,17] This disparity can lead to inaccurate assessment and inadequate management of anxiety in critically ill patients. Anxiety is defined as a feeling of uneasiness, discomfort, or dread[18]; therefore, it follows that an individual is the only one who can accurately describe what he or she may be feeling.

Several studies have been done to evaluate different tools that can be used to accurately assess anxiety in critically ill patients. The Faces Anxiety Scale has been identified as a valid measure of anxiety for nonverbal patients who are critically ill.[1] In a review of 10 different tools used to evaluate anxiety, Perpina-Galvan and Richart-Martinez[2] reported that patients have difficulty recognizing the face that correlates with the level of anxiety. In all tools that were reviewed, patients required help in completing the assessment. Of all the instruments evaluated, the recommended options for evaluating anxiety in critically ill patients are the Brief Symptoms Inventory (BSI-a) and the State Trait Anxiety Inventory (STAI-s). Both of these scales have 6 items, are easy to use and interpret, and have good reliability. Another potentially useful and simple tool is the 0 to 10 numeric rating scale that has been used extensively for reporting pain, although this tool has not been investigated for use with anxiety. In assessing levels of anxiety, it is also important for the nurse to remember cultural implications, as the norms and values of different cultures can affect the patient's perspective of anxiety or his or her willingness to report it as well as other manifestations.[4,19]

Accurate assessment of family anxiety is important as well because anxiety among family members can have a negative impact on their abilities to process and understand information, maintain normal family functioning, cope effectively, and provide support for patients and each other. It is also important to remember that the term "family" now means anyone who considers themselves a family member, as approximately one-third of families in this country are composed of members who have no biologic or legal relationship. Family anxiety may manifest as distrust of hospital staff, including health care providers, noncompliance with treatment, anger, complaints about care, or legal claims. Astute nursing assessment can facilitate early identification of potential problems of this nature and appropriate interventions to prevent and/or alleviate this type of anxiety to facilitate the most optimal outcomes for patients and families.[3]

NURSING DIAGNOSIS

Anxiety in critically ill patients is related to a variety of environmental factors. Examples include unfamiliar and frightening noises, constant light, painful procedures, situational crisis, threat of death, change in health status, and/or stress. Environmental factors are most clearly identified through the patient's self-report. Potential manifestations found in assessments include elevations in heart rate, respiratory rate, and blood pressure, as well as restlessness, agitation, need for attention, and seeking reassurance.[15] Still other manifestations include but are not limited to fidgeting, extraneous movements, fear, focus on self, wariness, irritability, tremors, facial tension, trembling, anorexia, diarrhea, and sleep disturbances.[18]

INTERVENTIONS

Studies indicate that medication administration in the form of sedatives and/or opioids is the primary intervention used by critical care nurses for alleviating anxiety especially in patients who require intubation and mechanical ventilation.[2,15,20] **Table 1** outlines the more commonly used medications for anxiety, sedation, and pain management, including classification, common dosages, and specific nursing responsibilities.[21–23] Some of the most commonly used medications are morphine, midazolam, and propofol. A recent study of 174 intensive care units including more than 100,000 mechanically ventilated patients over a 6-year period revealed that propofol is the most commonly used drug for sedation in these patients.[24] Other drugs sometimes used include diazepam, fentanyl, haloperidol, lorazepam, and meperidine. Assessment of the level of sedation is necessary when administering any of these drugs. Scales such as the Observer's Assessment of Alertness/Sedation is useful for assessing sedation with opioids, whereas scales such as the Ramsey Sedation Scale or the Richmond Agitation-Sedation Scale is useful for evaluating a patient's need for sedation.[25]

Although medications are essential components in the management of anxiety, studies indicate that despite administration of these drugs, as many as 34% of patients in critical care settings continue to experience moderate to severe anxiety,[1] with high levels of anxiety reported in those patients requiring mechanical ventilation.[2] There are many additional interventions that can be used by critical care nurses to help alleviate this level of anxiety and have a positive impact on patient outcomes.

In caring for any patient who is experiencing anxiety, critical care nurses must first establish a trusting therapeutic relationship with patients and their families with an attitude of empathy and concern for the patient's well-being. Critical care nurses must also be aware of their own levels of anxiety, which may contribute to the patient's level

Table 1
Medications used for anxiety in critical care

Lorazepam (Ativan)	
Classification	Benzodiazepine, sedative/hypnotic, anxiolytic
Dosage	IVP: 0.02–0.06 mg/kg every 2–6 hours at a rate of 2 mg/min (dilute in equal amount of sterile water, saline or 5% dextrose solution) IV infusion: 0.01–0.1 mg/kg/h No more than 5 mg/h USE FILTER
Adverse effects	Hypotension, tachycardia, rash, laryngospasm, confusion, apnea, bradypnea, bradycardia, somnolence
Nursing responsibilities	• Expect onset of action in less than 5 minutes with peak in 15–20 minutes. • Use smaller doses in the elderly to prevent hypotension. • Should be administered in large vein with continuous monitoring of vital signs during titration. • Elevate foot of bed and increase IV fluids in the event of severe hypotension. • Abrupt withdrawal can cause seizures. Antidote: flumazenil Not removed by hemodialysis
Midazolam (Versed)	
Classification	Benzodiazepine, sedative/hypnotic
Dosage	IVP: 0.02–0.08 mg/kg every 5–15 minutes each dose over 2 minutes undiluted IV infusion: 0.04–0.2 mg/kg/h up to 10 mg/h
Adverse effects	Hiccups, bradycardia, hypotension, drowsiness, respiratory depression, amnesia
Nursing responsibilities	• Elderly patients may require lower doses. • Continuous monitoring of vital signs is required. Be alert for paradoxic response—agitation. Abrupt withdrawal may cause seizures. Antidote: flumazenil Not removed by hemodialysis
Propofol (Diprivan)	
Classification	Anesthetic, sedative/hypnotic
Dosage	IV infusion: Start at 5 µg/kg/min for 5 minutes titrating up in 5–10 µg/kg/min increments up to maximum dose of 75 µg/kg/min
Adverse effects	Nausea, vomiting, fever, hypotension, apnea, bradycardia, cough, flushing, abdominal cramps

Nursing responsibilities	• Consider an 80% dosage reduction in the elderly.
	• Avoid in patients with increased intracranial pressure.
	• Avoid in children.
	• Abrupt discontinuation can result in rapid awakening, anxiety, agitation, resistance to mechanical ventilation.
	• Titrate dose down slowly—5 minutes between dosage adjustments.
	• Turns urine green.
	• Monitor BP every 15 minutes during titration, then every hour.
	• Continuous monitoring of HR, RR, SpO2, ECG.
	• Give atropine for bradycardia and IV fluids for hypotension along with down-titration of propofol.
	• If administered longer than 48 hours, implement sedation vacation each day to assess neurologic status.
	• Onset of action is 30 seconds with duration of 3–10 minutes.
	• Must use facility-approved Sedation Scale for documentation of sedation level every 4 hours.
	• Change IV tubing every 12 hours. IV push dosing and administration to a nonintubated patient is NOT within the scope of practice for the RN and may only be administered by persons trained in the administration of anesthesia.

Morphine sulfate

Classification	Opioid narcotic analgesic
Dosage	IVP: 1–2 mg every hour as needed; may be given undiluted over 5 minutes
	IV infusion: 0.8–10 mg/h up to 80 mg/h
Adverse effects	Sedation, hypotension, diaphoresis, facial flushing, constipation, nausea, vomiting, dizziness, somnolence, respiratory depression, urinary retention
Nursing responsibilities	• Adverse effects markedly increased with rapid administration.
	• Patient should be supine during administration. Reduce dose for elderly or debilitated patients.
	• Use extreme caution in patients with preexisting hypotension, respiratory depression, renal impairment, or hepatic impairment.
	• Continuous monitoring of vital signs, including pulse oximetry if continuous infusion is used.
	• Hold the drug for respiratory rate less than 9 breaths/minute unless mechanical ventilation is in use or in the case of comfort care only.
	• Elderly patients in particular should have a stool softener or laxative ordered as constipation is very common.
	• Pain assessment should occur before administration of each IVP dose and within 5 minutes after, as onset of action is rapid with peak action at 20 minutes.
	• Patients should be comfortable with a pain level of no more than 3 on a 0 to 10 scale.

Abbreviations: ECG, electrocardiogram; HR, heart rate; IV, intravenous; IVP, IV push; RR, respiratory rate; SpO₂, pulse oximetry.

Data from Algozzine G, Algozzine R, Lilly D. Critical care intravenous infusion drug handbook. 3rd edition. St Louis: Elsevier; 2010; Baird M, Bridgers C, Schmidt P. Mosby's critical care drug reference. St Louis: Elsevier; 2008; and Clinical clue: who administers propofol? AACN: Bold Voices 2009;1(2):9.

of anxiety. It is imperative that nurses maintain a calm, reassuring approach using a controlled, soothing voice when interacting with patients and families. Simply being available to listen and talk can be an effective tool for alleviating high levels of anxiety. It is important for nurses to acknowledge the patient's anxiety, encouraging expression of feelings and to provide reality-based information without giving false hope. Critical care nurses must also recognize that anxiety is a normal response to certain situations that may provide a means of coping for the individual until such time that the reality of a situation can be processed and accepted. A patient who has just been given the news of a cancer diagnosis may use denial as a means of coping until the diagnosis can be accepted. The patient should be encouraged to use anxiety in coping with such situations if helpful, as a moderate level of anxiety can sharpen awareness and help the client to focus on dealing with the problem. During high levels of anxiety, it is important for the nurse to remain with the patient using a calm, confident manner and speaking in brief, simple terms.[26]

For anxiety that is specifically related to fear of death and dying, in addition to pain control,[27] it is very important to provide opportunities for the patient and family to verbalize their fears and respond to these fears in a caring and supportive way.[28] Additionally, it may helpful to assist patients with a life review while providing a supportive and nurturing environment with open and honest communication about the patient's prognosis based on his or her level of acceptance of the situation.[29] Some find relief of anxiety through spiritual means. Given it is an acceptable measure, encouraging the patient and family to pray and providing for visitation and support from a personal minister or hospital chaplain can also provide comfort at the end of life.[30] Allowing self-determination about end-of-life decisions when possible can also provide a means of control for the patient and afford some relief to family members about making those difficult decisions.

Nurses should use empathy to encourage the patient to see the anxiety as a normal response to the stressors present in the current environment. This response will help to validate the patient's feelings and promote a sense of well-being.[31] If the patient is experiencing thoughts or fears that are irrational, nurses should provide accurate information and encourage patients to discuss the meaning of the events that are contributing to the feelings of anxiety.[19] Talking about the perceived threats may be all that is necessary to alleviate a great deal of anxiety; however, nurses should intervene whenever possible to remove the source of anxiety.[19] Because anxiety is a normal response to actual or perceived danger, if the threat is removed, the response ceases. Interventions such as responding quickly to ventilator alarms, cardiac-monitoring alarms, infusion pump alarms, and call lights can effectively alleviate a rise in anxiety.

All activities and procedures, including potential sensory reactions, should be explained in simple terms to promote understanding before implementing procedures or even touching the patient.[32–37] For example, when preparing patients for endotracheal suctioning, warning of the sensation to need to cough as a normal response that will resolve with completion of the procedure and providing reassurance that oxygenation is being maintained can help patients to realize that there is an end to the uncomfortable nature of the procedure. Also, letting patients know that the suction attempt will last no longer than 10 seconds can assure an individual that the procedure will end shortly and he or she will be comfortable again. Simple procedures such as repositioning may instill fear and should be explained in advance, as should other potentially painful procedures, such as blood draws, wound care, dressing changes, and even mouth care for patients who are intubated.

There is a significant amount of evidence to indicate that listening to music is effective for decreasing anxiety in several different populations of critically ill patients.

Evidence indicates that a single music therapy session is effective for decreasing anxiety in patients who are mechanically ventilated[38,39] as indicated by improvement in heart rate and respiratory rate. Numerous other studies support the use of music in a variety of critically ill patients for reducing anxiety.[40–46] Evidence indicates that the most important factor in facilitating relaxation is to focus on types of music that are desirable to the patient.[47] Although patient preference is the most important determinant for music selection, White[45] documented that slow, repetitive, steady rhythms seem to have the most soothing effect on the listener.

Other comfort measures might include short massages of the back, feet, and/or hands.[48–50] Family members may be encouraged to become involved in this intervention as well. Nurses can teach family members the proper technique for massaging the hands, feet, and/or back, which can provide feelings of usefulness and decrease the sense of helplessness for the family as well as to provide some relief of anxiety for the patients and families.[51]

Although important for all ages, it is especially important for nurses to provide a safe and protective environment for geriatric patients. This can be done by maintaining consistent caregivers and the typical environmental structure.[19] Also important in this endeavor is responding to alarms in a timely manner. Explaining the reason for these alarms and responding quickly will help to alleviate anxiety related to the fear that the alarms indicate an emergent change in the patient's condition. Critical care nurses should discuss safety precautions that are used with ventilator support, such as the availability of an emergency power source and emergency oxygen equipment. Patients should be assured that the call light is within easy reach at all times and if necessary an alternative means of calling for assistance should be provided.[52]

Maintaining a quiet environment can also decrease anxiety, as excessive noise results in sensory overload resulting in an increase in anxiety.[6] Maintaining an awareness of the effects of loud conversations outside the patient's room and even customary interactions of numerous health care providers can help to alleviate anxiety related to excessive noise. Keeping the patient's door closed if closed circuit video provides a means of surveillance is a simple way to decrease unnecessary noise. Attention to details such as reducing the constant use of artificial lighting and opening windows during the day for natural light can help to enhance pain management, decrease depression, and improve the quality of sleep.[6]

EXPECTED OUTCOMES

Expected outcomes related to patient improvement include identifying and reporting anxiety using a numeric rating scale or the Faces Anxiety Scale. It is equally important to elicit at least one technique identified by the patient for controlling anxiety. Outcomes of interventions include a decrease in distress as manifested by vital signs that reflect a decrease in sympathetic nervous system activity and patient display of a relaxed posture and facial expression as well as gestures and activity levels that reflect a decrease in distress.[19]

FAMILY INTERVENTION

Providing care for the families of critically ill patients is also important, as critical illness affects all members of the family unit. A holistic approach to care includes the family in the plan of care when possible to increase their feelings of overall satisfaction with the experience and allay anxiety. Needs of families have been categorized as receiving assurance, remaining near the patient, receiving information, being comfortable, and having support available.[3]

When families are dissatisfied with care, the most common complaint is lack of communication.[6] To meet the need for information, nurses must begin communication early with family members to present a caring, concerned attitude to establish a trusting relationship. Informing families that they will be kept informed at regular intervals and have opportunities to ask questions and express concerns is a crucial aspect of family care. Providing daily reports about changes in the patient's condition in nonmedical jargon at specified times helps to reassure the family that the nurse is also concerned about their well-being. Because the critical care environment may be intimidating and frightening, talking with families before they enter the unit for the first time is a critical step in allaying anxiety and fear. An explanation of sounds such as ventilator alarms, cardiac monitor alarms, and infusion pump alarms can help to alleviate some of the initial anxiety. Also, assuring the family that most alarms are not indicative of an emergency and responding to alarms quickly indicates that the nurses are vigilant in providing safe care. Also, an explanation of the appearance of the patient along with any equipment being used in the patient's care can help to prepare the family for a potentially frightening first visit.

Effective communication as it relates to end-of-life care is also important in providing a positive experience as much as possible for dying patients and their families. Clear and consistent communication from all members of the health care team about the patient's prognosis as well as the plan of care and allowing family members to express grief and concern is helpful in increasing satisfaction with care and facilitating more positive bereavement. Decisions regarding the level of care to be provided should include family, physicians, nurses, and most of all, the patient when possible. If the patient is unable to participate in decision making, a current living will or durable power of attorney should be used to represent the patient's wishes about treatment toward the end of life. It is also important for the family to feel confident that the patient will not be abandoned when aggressive care measures are replaced with palliative care in the event that aggressive measures are deemed futile.[53] As stress can affect the family's memory of information, a brief written guide for the family is helpful in reinforcing needed information (**Table 2**).

Open visitation is another strategy for meeting the need to be in close proximity to the patient. Numerous studies have shown that open visitation produces no deleterious effects to the patient or family[54] but can actually have a positive impact on the patient's condition.[55] Some intensive care units have extended open visitation to include children and pets.[6] In addition, allowing a family member to remain with the patient may alleviate anxiety for the patient and family member alike. Open visitation not only enables families to remain near their loved one but has a positive impact on the satisfaction of the patient and family regarding the critical care experience and quality of care. It also provides opportunities for the nurses to provide information, reassurance, and support. If open visitation is not an option, a good substitute is a waiting room that is in close proximity to the ICU, so that the family members remain near the patient. The addition of pillows, blankets, and comfortable seating and refreshment opportunities can provide additional comfort.

Recent research[56] shows that family members who are invited to participate in the fundamental care of patients perceive an increase in respect, collaboration, and overall family-centered care than those family members who are not invited to participate in fundamental care. The most common care activities that family members provided in this study were massage, bathing, and eye care. Other care activities included hair combing, mouth care, face wash, hair wash, shave, antithrombotic stockings

Table 2 Family guide for ICU
Doctor's Name
Nurse's Name
Patient's Diagnosis
Unit Phone Number
Visiting Hours
Approximate Time for Doctor's Visit
Location of Cafeteria/Restrooms
The Critical Care Environment: • There are numerous unfamiliar noises that you will hear in the ICU, such as ventilator (breathing machine) noises, ventilator alarms, heart monitor alarms, alarms for equipment used for giving fluids through the veins, and alarms for equipment used for giving food through a tube. • These alarms serve to alert the nurse to check on the patient—most alarms do not indicate a serious change in your family member's condition. • The nurse will respond to these alarms quickly to correct any problem. • Your nurse will talk with you at least once during each shift as well as any time there is a change in the patient's condition. • If you think of questions, it is a good idea to write them down, as it is easy to forget during this stressful time. Things you can do to help: • Talk to your loved one when visiting in a calm manner. • Tell her/him the day, time, and nonstressful news from home. Feel free to touch the person and reassure him/her that you are present. • The nurse might also ask you help with bathing, exercises, or repositioning your loved one. • Ask the nurse how you can help if you would like to participate in the care of your loved one. • Please be aware that if you are sick with a cold, the flu, or other infections, exposing your loved one to these illnesses could make his/her condition worse. • Please use hand sanitizer upon entering and leaving the patient's room for your protection and the patient's protection.

application, and limb exercises. Nurses can assess family members' comfort with and desire to provide care as well as determine appropriate care for them to provide depending on individual patients' needs and family member abilities. Supporting family participation in fundamental care provides an opportunity for the family members to remain close to the patient and feel useful and promotes a healthy work environment with collaboration of care. Providing this type of support for family members can decrease their levels of anxiety and facilitate their coping abilities.[57]

Some institutions have implemented a policy for family presence during cardiopulmonary resuscitation (CPR) and invasive procedures, as studies have shown a potential decrease in anxiety and fear.[58] Other benefits include a sense of closure and initiation of more positive grieving, being with and supporting their loved one, feeling that everything possible was done, and removing doubt about the patient's condition. Allowing family presence supports a more holistic approach and family-centered care especially during CPR.[59] Duran[55] reports that families feel that they have a right to be present and would like the option to be offered to them. Families surveyed reported that being present during these types of events was helpful and that they could control their emotions. Overall, health care providers are supportive despite some concerns for the safety of patients and families, as well as their emotional well-being and performance anxiety. Family presence during any type of medical intervention should be based on individual situation and family desires. When implementing this practice, it is important to remember that someone should be designated to remain with the family to provide support, answer questions, and provide explanations during resuscitation efforts. If resuscitation efforts are unsuccessful, a time for debriefing should occur as soon as possible after the event. Ideally, a nurse with psychology and mental health preparation could be available to assist with this component of family care. Collaboration with a psychology and mental health nurse can also be helpful in accurate assessment and appropriate interventions for controlling anxiety in critically ill patients, as they are well versed in recognizing manifestations that may not otherwise be recognized as indicators of anxiety.

SUMMARY

Critical care nurses are at the bedside of critically ill patients around the clock and have the greatest opportunity to have an impact on outcomes for these patients and their families. As anxiety for these patients presents an opportunity of increased risks for morbidity and mortality, it is imperative that nurses strive to identify unrelieved anxiety early to prevent adverse events. Accurate assessment, safe medication administration, effective communication, environmental controls, comfort measures, flexibility, vigilance, and a supportive attitude provide a foundation for success in meeting the needs of patients and families suffering from anxiety as a result of the critical care experience.

REFERENCES

1. McKinley S, Stein-Parbury J, Chehelnabi A, et al. Assessment of anxiety in intensive care patients by using the faces anxiety scale. Am J Crit Care 2004;13(2): 146–52.
2. Perpina-Galvan J, Richart-Martinez M. Scales for evaluating self-perceived anxiety levels in patients admitted to intensive care units: a review. Am J Crit Care 2009;18(6):571–80.
3. Leske JS. Interventions to decrease family anxiety. Crit Care Nurse 2002;22(6): 61–5.
4. Chan KS, Twinn S. An analysis of the stressors and coping strategies of Chinese adults with a partner admitted to an intensive care unit in Hong Kong: an exploratory study. J Clin Nurs 2006;16:185–93.
5. Frazier SK, Moser DK, Riegel B, et al. Critical care nurses' assessment of patients' anxiety: reliance on physiological and behavioral parameters. Am J Crit Care 2002;11(1):57–64.
6. Hosmanek M, Sole JL. The critical care experience. In: Sole ML, Klein DG, Moseley MJ, editors. Introduction to critical care nursing. 5th edition. St Louis (MO): Mosby; 2009. p. 11–25.
7. Novaes MA, Aronovich A, Ferraz MB, et al. Stressors in ICU: patients' evaluation. Intensive Care Med 1997;23:1282–5.
8. Antai-Onong D. The client with an anxiety disorder. In: Psychiatric nursing: biological and behavioral concepts. New York: Delmar; 2008. p. 297–341.
9. Frasure-Smith N. In-hospital symptoms of psychological stress as predictors of long-term outcome after acute myocardial infarction in men. Am J Cardiol 1991;67:121–7.
10. Kiecolt-Glaser JK, Marucha PT, Malarkey WB, et al. Slowing of wound healing by psychological stress. Lancet 1995;346:1194–6.

11. Moser DK, Dracup K. Is anxiety early after myocardial infarction associated with subsequent ischemic and arrhythmic events? Psychosom Med 1996;58: 395–401.

12. Priori SG, Zuanetti G, Schwartz PJ. Ventricular fibrillation induced by the interaction between acute myocardial ischemia and sympathetic hyperactivity: effect of nifedipine. Am Heart J 1988;116:37–43.

13. Rozanski A, Krantz DS, Bairey CN. Ventricular response to mental stress testing in patients with coronary artery disease: pathophysiologic implications. Circulation 1991;83(Suppl):137–44.

14. Travazzi L, Zotti AM, Rondanelli R. The role of psychologic stress in the genesis of lethal arrhythmias in patients with coronary artery disease. Eur Heart J 1986;7 (Suppl):99–106.

15. Moser DK, Chung ML, McKinley S, et al. Critical care nursing practice regarding patient anxiety assessment and management. Intensive Crit Care Nurs 2003;19: 276–88.

16. O'Brien JL, Moser DK, Reigel B, et al. Comparison of anxiety assessments between clinicians and patients with acute MI in cardiac critical care units. Am J Crit Care 2001;10:97–103.

17. Van der Dores A. Patients' and nurses' rating of pain and anxiety during burn wound care. Pain 1989;39:95–101.

18. Neal MC, editor. Nursing diagnosis: definition and classification. Philadelphia: NANDA International; 2007. p. 9–10.

19. McCaffrey R. Anxiety. In: Ackley BJ, Ladwig GB, editors. Nursing diagnosis handbook. 8th edition. St Louis (MO): Mosby; 2008. p. 139–44.

20. Frazier SK, Moser DK, Daley LK, et al. Critical care nurses' beliefs about and reported management of anxiety. Am J Crit Care 2003;12(1):19–27.

21. Algozzine G, Algozzine R, Lilly D. Critical care intravenous infusion drug handbook. 3rd edition. St Louis (MO): Elsevier; 2010.

22. Baird M, Bridgers C, Schmidt P. Mosby's citical care drug reference. St Louis (MO): Elsevier; 2008.

23. Clinical Clue: who administers propofol? AACN: Bold Voices 2009;1(2):9.

24. Wunsch H, Kahn J, Kramer A, et al. Use of intravenous infusion sedation among mechanically ventilated patients in the United States. Crit Care Med;37(12): 3031–9.

25. Li D, Puntillo K. Ask the experts. Crit Care Nurse 2004;24(1):68–72.

26. Doenges ME, Moorhouse MF, Murr AC. Nurse's pocket guide: diagnoses, prioritized interventions, and rationales. 10th edition. Philadelphia: FA Davis; 2006. p. 82–7.

27. Deffner J, Bell S. Nurses' death anxiety, comfort level during communication with patients and families regarding death, and exposure to communication education: a quantitative study. J Nurses Staff Dev 2005;21(1):19–23.

28. Dunne K. Effective communication in palliative care. Nurs Stand 2005;20(13): 57–64.

29. Heyland D, Dodek P, Groll D, et al. What matters most in end-of-life care: perceptions of seriously ill patients and their family members. CMAJ 2006;174(5):627–33.

30. Forbes MA, Rosdahl DR. The final journey of life. J Hosp Palliat Nurs 2003;5(4): 213–20.

31. Alasad J, Ahmad M. Communication with critically ill patients. J Adv Nurs 2005;50(3):256–62.

32. Gallaher R, McKinley S. Stressors and anxiety in patients undergoing coronary artery bypass surgery. Am J Crit Care 2007;16(3):248–57.

33. Johnson JE. Effects of structuring patients' expectations on their reactions to threatening events. Nurs Res 1972;21:499–504.

34. Kim H, Garvin BJ, Moser DK. Stress during mechanical ventilation: benefit of having concrete objective information before cardiac surgery. Am J Crit Care 1999;8:118–26.

35. Kisely S, Simon G. An international study comparing the effect of medically explained and unexplained somatic symptoms on psychosocial outcome. J Psychosom Res 2006;60(2):125–30.

36. Shi SF, Munjas BA, Wan TT, et al. The effects of preparatory sensory information on ICU patients. J Med Syst 2003;27:191–204.

37. Suls J, Wan CK. Effects of sensory and procedural information on coping with stressful medical procedures and pain: a meta analysis. J Consult Clin Psychol 1989;57:372–9.

38. Chlan L. Music therapy as a nursing intervention for patients supported by mechanical ventilation. AACN Clin Issues 2000;11(1):128–38.

39. Chlan L. The effectiveness of a music therapy intervention on relaxation and anxiety for patients receiving ventilator assistance. Heart Lung 1998;27:169–76.

40. Barnason S, Zimmerman L, Nieveen J. The effect of music interventions on anxiety in the patient after coronary artery bypass grafting. Heart Lung 1995; 24:124–32.

41. Elliott D. The effects of music and muscle relaxation on patient anxiety in a coronary care unit. Heart Lung 1994;23:27–35.

42. Guzzetta CE. Effects of relaxation and music therapy on patients in a coronary care unit with presumptive acute myocardial infarction. Heart Lung 1989;18: 609–16.

43. Krucoff MW, Crater SW, Gallup D, et al. Music, imagery, touch, and prayer as adjuncts to interventional cardiac care: the Monitoring and Actualization of Noetic Trainings (MANTRA) II randomized study. Lancet 2005;366(9481):211–7.

44. Twiss E, Seaver J, McCaffrey R. The effect of music listening on anxiety and post-operative ventilation in older adults undergoing cardiovascular surgery. Nurs Crit Care 2006;23(5):245–51.

45. White JM. State of the science of music interventions: critical care and perioperative practice. Crit Care Nurs Clin North Am 2000;12(2):219–25.

46. Wong HL, Lopez-Nahas V, Molassiotis A. Effects of music therapy on anxiety in ventilator-dependent patients. Heart Lung 2000;30:376–87.

47. Stratton VN, Zalanowski AH. The relationship between music, degree of liking, and self-reported relaxation. J Music Ther 1984;21:184–92.

48. Hayes J, Cox C. Immediate effects of a five minute foot massage on patients in critical care. Intensive Crit Care Nurs 1999;15:77–82.

49. Keegan L. Alternative and complementary modalities for managing stress and anxiety. Crit Care Nurse 2003;23:55–8.

50. Mok E, Woo CP. The effects of slow-stroke back massage on anxiety and pain in elderly stroke patients. Complement Ther Nurs Midwifery 2004;10(4):209–16.

51. Jansen MPM, Schmitt NA. Family-focused interventions. Crit Care Nurs Clin North Am 2003;15:347–54.

52. Comer S. Delmar's critical care nursing care plans. 2nd edition. Clifton Park (NY): Thompson Delmar Learning; 2005. p. 98.

53. Houghton D. End-of-life care in the critical care unit. In: Sole ML, Klein DG, Moseley MJ, editors. Introduction to critical care nursing. 5th edition. St Louis (MO): Mosby; 2009. p. 43–52.

54. Roland P, Russell J, Richards KC, et al. Visitation in critical care: processes and outcomes of a performance improvement initiative. J Nurs Care Qual 2001;15(2): 18–26.
55. Duran CR, Oman KS, Abel JJ, et al. Attitudes toward and beliefs about family presence: a survey of healthcare providers, patients' families, and patients. Am J Crit Care 2007;16(3):270–9.
56. Mitchell M, Chaboyer W, Burmeister E, et al. Positive effects of a nursing intervention on family-centered care in adult critical care. Am J Crit Care 2009;18(6): 543–53.
57. Mitchell ML, Courtney M. Reducing family members' anxiety and uncertainty in illness around transfer from intensive care: an intervention study. Intensive Crit Care Nurs 2004;20(4):223–31.
58. Halm MA. Family presence during resuscitation: a critical review of the literature. Am J Crit Care 2005;14(6):494–512.
59. Baumhover N, Hughes L. Spirituality and support for family presence during invasive procedures and resuscitations in adults. Am J Crit Care 2009;18(4): 357–67.

Traumatic Brain Injury in Operation Enduring Freedom/ Operation Iraqi Freedom: A Primer

Katherine S. Fabrizio, PhD[a],*, Norman L. Keltner, EdD, CRNP[b]

KEYWORDS

• Brain injury • Blast • Military • Veterans

Approximately 1.64 million service members have been deployed as a part of Operation Enduring Freedom (OEF) and Operation Iraqi Freedom (OIF) since September 2001.[1] Fortunately, improvements in trauma care in the battlefield and advances in protective equipment have resulted in higher numbers of service members who are able to survive injuries that would have been fatal in the past.[2,3] Even so, changes in warfare through the increased use of explosive devices have resulted in service members who are at increased risk for injury when compared with rates from prior conflicts.[3,4] It is estimated that approximately 19.5% of the service members who have served as part of OEF/OIF have sustained a probable traumatic brain injury (TBI) during deployment, which is equivalent to approximately 320,000 service members.[1] It is imperative that health care profession professionals gain a better understanding of the injuries faced by service members, because their injuries are likely to result in lifelong care needs.

Although a vast amount of literature exists regarding TBIs in the civilian population, the literature regarding TBI in the military is less robust. This article will focus on the basics of TBI, with an emphasis on the types of injuries that are typically sustained in combat. The impact of post-traumatic stress disorder (PTSD) in the TBI population will be discussed. Treatments will be explored, with an emphasis on the pharmacologic treatments commonly employed by nurses. Finally, two case studies of veterans who sustained combat TBIs will be presented.

[a] Physical Medicine and Rehabilitation (117), Birmingham Veterans Affairs Medical Center, 700 South 19th Street, Birmingham, AL 35233, USA
[b] University of Alabama School of Nursing, University of Alabama at Birmingham, 1701 University Boulevard, Birmingham, AL 35294, USA
* Corresponding author.
E-mail address: Katherine.Fabrizio@va.gov

Nurs Clin N Am 45 (2010) 569–580
doi:10.1016/j.cnur.2010.06.003
0029-6465/10/$ – see front matter. Published by Elsevier Inc.

nursing.theclinics.com

TRAUMATIC BRAIN INJURY: INTRODUCTION

A brain injury, simply defined, is any trauma to the brain that is sustained through blunt force, penetration of the skull, or acceleration/deceleration of the brain. Typically, the injuries are divided into two categories: open and closed injuries. An open-head injury includes trauma in which the skull is penetrated by an object, such as a bullet or projectile, or when fragments of the skull are depressed into the brain. People with open-head injuries may not lose consciousness, and they may present with focal deficits that correspond with the lesion area. In contrast, a closed-head injury results from a blow to the head, without penetration of the skull (although the skull can be damaged). Closed-head injuries are the most common type of brain injury and will be the focus of this article.

Several events are set into motion as soon as the brain is injured. The brain, which is surrounded by fluid, moves within the skull because of the forces sustained during the injury. There can be a rapid acceleration and deceleration of the brain, as well as rotational forces, which place stress on the brain. The strain on the neurons caused by the rapid changes in force also can result in tearing and shearing of axons, known as diffuse axonal injury. In closed-head injuries, the frontal and temporal lobes are particularly vulnerable to damage because of the boney protrusions on the inside of the skull in those regions.

Following the injury, a cascade of physiologic events then begins. These events can be equal to or in some cases greater than the destructive effects previously described.[5,6] Increased fluid collection with swelling (edema) and bruising (hemorrhaging) also may occur and lead to further compromise. Metabolic changes in levels of potassium and calcium, as well as changes in glucose metabolism, also begin and can lead to cell death.[7]

Information about the initial injury serves as a useful predictor of the extent to which the brain will experience the previously described events. Severity of TBI also can provide clues as to the overall predicted outcome and potential deficits. Determination of TBI severity is based on several factors, including the patient's level of arousal/consciousness at the time of injury, the duration of the loss of consciousness (LOC), and the duration of post-traumatic amnesia (PTA, the length of memory disruption following injury). The Glasgow Coma Scale (GCS) is an assessment tool that measures level of consciousness and arousal, with a score of 15 indicating normal arousal and orientation (**Table 1**).[8]

A caveat about the GCS is that it can be influenced by many factors, including how long post-injury the assessment is conducted and presence of medications/drugs at time of measurement.[9] It has been suggested that PTA is the best predictor of injury severity.[10,11] Generally, the period of PTA ends when the patient begins to continuously register experiences. Clinically, this could manifest as knowledge from the patient that an injury has occurred and demonstrated awareness of hospitalization.

There is often some variation in the metrics used to define injury severity, but one commonly used classification system is shown in **Table 2**. Specifics about all three factors (GCS, LOC, and PTA) need not be known to classify TBI severity.

TBI IN THE COMBAT THEATER

Within the combat theater, a service member is exposed to many of the same causes of TBI as in the civilian world, such as falls and motor vehicle accidents (MVAs). In the OEF/OIF conflict, however, there has been widespread use of explosive devices, including improvised explosive devices (IEDs or roadside bombs), rocket-propelled grenades, mortars, and artillery, thus exposing the service member to additional injury

Table 1
Glasgow Coma Scale

		Score
Motor	Obeys verbal commands	6
	Localizes to noxious stimuli	5
	Normal flexion to noxious stimuli	4
	Abnormal flexion to noxious stimuli (decorticate posturing)	3
	Extension to noxious stimuli (decerebrate posturing)	2
	No response to noxious stimuli	1
Verbal	Fully oriented and converses	5
	Disoriented and converses	4
	Voices appropriate words	3
	Makes incomprehensible sounds	2
	No vocalization	1
Eye Opening	Opens eyes spontaneously	4
	Opens eyes to verbal commands	3
	Opens eyes to noxious stimuli	2
	No eye opening	1
Total Score		3–15

mechanisms. In the current conflict, many service members are required to travel long distances by vehicle, placing them at risk for MVAs and exposure to IEDs. In addition to direct injuries from frequent mortar and rocket attacks, indirect injuries sustained when the service member is seeking cover also are reported.

The overall effect on the brain due to a blast injury is similar to that of other mechanisms, but there are four categories of blast-specific effects that can be sustained, including primary, secondary, tertiary, and quaternary.[12] The primary effects are the direct effects of the pressure wave to the air-filled organs (eg, tympanic membrane, lungs, colon, and eyes are the most commonly impacted), in which there is a rapid increase or decrease in pressure. Penetrating wounds caused by the fragments that are commonly contained in the explosive device comprise the secondary effects. The force of the blast may result in such a strong wind that the person is displaced or a structure collapses. Crush injuries and blunt trauma from these forces comprise the tertiary effects. Finally, quaternary effects include burns and injuries caused by inhalation of fumes, dust, or smoke.

Beyond the impact on the brain, blasts can result in numerous other injuries, including amputations, musculoskeletal injuries, spinal cord injuries, and mental health problems. Service members returning from combat with a disabling injury (one of which has to be life-threatening) to more than one region of the body are said to have experienced polytrauma. Common polytrauma injuries for OEF/OIF service members include TBI and post-traumatic stress disorder (PTSD). Researchers identified several common factors for service members sustaining a TBI during their OEF/OIF deployment,

Table 2
Traumatic brain injury severity classification

Severity of Traumatic Brain Injury	Glasgow Coma Scale	Duration of Loss of Consciousness	Duration of Post-traumatic Amnesia
Mild	13–15	0–30 minutes	<24 hours
Moderate	8–12	30 minutes-24 hours	>24 hours
Severe	3–8	>24 hours	>7 days

compared with service members who are injured but do not experience a TBI.[13] Those factors include: engagement in high combat intensity, injury by a blast, exposure to more than one explosion, younger age, lower rank, and male gender.[13]

Preliminary data on the prevalence of TBI in the military population revealed that, of the total number of TBIs, approximately half were mild in severity.[3] Anecdotally, within Veterans Administration (VA) hospitals, most injuries treated are mild in severity, with fewer veterans presenting with moderate-to-severe combat-related TBIs. It has been suggested that most of those who experience a mild TBI (mTBI) will make a good recovery.[2] For a portion of those who experience mTBI, however, persistent symptoms remain. Symptoms including headaches, dizziness, sensitivity to light, irritability, difficulty concentrating, and fatigue may be present months, even years, following the original injury. A complicating factor in the assessment and treatment of mTBI is that many of the symptoms of persistent sequelae of mTBI overlap with psychiatric disorders, such as PTSD. Shared symptoms include insomnia, irritability/anger, and trouble concentrating.[14]

ASSESSMENT OF TBI IN THE VETERAN POPULATION

To improve assessment and allow for triaging of service members upon returning from combat, the VA has implemented several clinical reminders designed specifically to address issues common to those who served as part of OEF/OIF. Clinical reminders, which are a series of questions the veteran is asked by a provider, address common concerns, including PTSD, depression, alcohol abuse, and suicidality. Currently, when a veteran who served in combat after Sept. 11, 2001, presents to the VA, he or she is asked a series of four questions to determine the possibility of a TBI and the current symptoms (**Box 1**). A positive screen is obtained when a veteran answers yes to all four of the questions. These screening questions were first implemented in April 2007.

Once identified as having a possible brain injury (by obtaining a positive screen), the veteran is then referred to the Traumatic Brain Injury Clinic for further assessment and treatment. A trained clinician completes a thorough history and physical examination, with an emphasis placed on a description of the possible TBI-producing event/s and the current symptoms. An algorithm is followed, and the appropriate treatment is initiated. Referrals to specialists, such as neurology for seizure management, neuropsychology for a detailed cognitive assessment, and speech therapy for cognitive treatment, are made. Because mood factors are often present, mental health treatment is an important part of treatment of TBI in the veteran population.

TBI SEQUELAE

It is challenging to describe the typical symptoms seen after a TBI, as there are vast differences depending on location, type, and severity of injury. Furthermore, recovery time can be a matter of hours for a mild injury to years for a severe injury and may include numerous conditions that are beyond the scope of this article. Therefore, the focus here is on cognitive and emotional/behavioral symptoms that may accompany the injury. **Table 3** outlines the cognitive and emotional symptoms that have been consistently reported in the literature.

Cognitive deficits vary significantly depending on the severity of the injury, but can include disruptions in processing speed, attention, memory, sensory/motor functioning, and executive skills.[15–20] Patients with slowed processing speed and attention problems may subjectively report difficulty thinking clearly, trouble completing tasks, and increased distractibility. At the more severe level, these problems could manifest

---

Box 1
VA TBI screening tool

During any of your OEF/OIF deployment(s), did you experience any of the following events? (check all that apply)

Blast or explosion (eg, IED, rocket-propelled grenade [RPG], land mine, grenade)

Vehicular accident/crash (any vehicles, including aircraft)

Fragment wound or bullet wound above the shoulders

Fall

Blow to the head (eg, hit head by falling/flying object, hit head by another person, hit head against something else)

Other injury to the head

Did you have any of the following symptoms immediately afterwards? (check all that apply)

Losing consciousness/knocked out

Being dazed, confused, or seeing stars

Not remembering the event

Concussion

Head injury

Did any of the following problems begin or get worse afterwards? (check all that apply)

Memory problems or lapses

Balance problems or dizziness

Sensitivity to bright light

Irritability

Headaches

Sleep problems

In the past week, have you had any of the symptoms from question 3? (check all that apply)

Memory problems or lapses

Balance problems or dizziness

Sensitivity to bright light

Irritability

Headaches

Sleep problems

---

as confusion and difficulty attending to a task for more than a few minutes. Memory deficits typically are caused by problems with acquisition and retrieval of information, with difficulty on memory recall tests.[18] Sensory and motor functioning problems typically impact only those with more severe injuries. These deficits include difficulty with reflexes, motor control, balance, and tone. Finally, impairments in executive (frontal) functions are often present in those with severe injuries. Clinically, this can manifest as inhibition of impulses, inappropriate behaviors, and a lack of insight into one's own abilities and deficits.

In addition to the cognitive effects, those with a TBI can experience mood changes. Research has suggested that there are two types of mood disorders that develop

Table 3	
Symptoms and syndromes associated with traumatic brain injury	
Cognitive	**Emotional and Behavioral**
Attention problems	Aggression
Executive dysfunction (planning, abstract reasoning, problem solving, insight, judgment)	Alcohol abuse
	Avolition
	Attention deficit hyperactivity disorder (ADHD)
Impaired judgment and decision making	Depression
Impaired self-awareness	Disinhibition
Memory problems	Irritability
Working memory problems	Post-traumatic stress disorder
Word-finding difficulties	Psychosis

Data from Jorge RE. Neuropsychiatric consequences of traumatic brain injury: a review of recent findings. Curr Opin Psychiatry 2005;18:289–99; Keltner NL, Cooke BB. Traumatic brain injury-war related. Perspect Psychiatr Care 2007;43(4):223–6; Kim E, Lauterbach EC, Reeve A, et al. Neuropsychiatric complications of traumatic brain injury: a critical review of the literature (a report of the ANPA Committee on Research). J Neuropsychiatry Clin Neurosci 2007;19(2):106–27; and Mathias JL, Wheaton P. Changes in attention and information-processing speed following severe traumatic brain injury: a meta-analytic review. Neuropsychology 2007;21:212–23.

following TBI: one that is based in the biologic changes in cortical and subcortical areas that are partially responsible for emotional processing, and one that is based in the psychological reaction to the sudden onset of disability.[21,22] Prevalence estimates indicate that depression following TBI is approximately 30%, while other mood disorders, such as mania, are less frequent.[23,24] In addition to depression and mania, PTSD can develop in response to the trauma that produced the TBI. Due to the prevalence of TBI and PTSD in the military population, a detailed discussion of this relationship is warranted.

PTSD AND TBI

PTSD, as defined by the *Diagnostic and Statistical Manual of Mental Disorders* (Fourth Edition) *DSM-IV*, requires

Exposure to an event that resulted in actual or threatened death of others, or threat to self;

The persistent re-experiencing (such as nightmares and flashbacks);

Persistent avoidance (such as avoidance of feelings, conversations, or activities that produce recollections of the trauma, estrangement from others, and restricted range of affect);

Persistent increased arousal (including insomnia, irritability, difficulty concentrating, and exaggerated startle response).

Symptoms must be present for greater than 3 months to receive the diagnosis of chronic PTSD.

One of the interesting discussions regarding PTSD and TBI is the question of whether these two diagnostic entities can co-exist. Those who favor a "no" response to the question make the convincing argument that since a cardinal symptom of PTSD is the remembering of the traumatic event, the diagnostic criteria for TBI renders the two diagnoses mutually exclusive phenomena. For example, key PTSD symptoms such as flashbacks, thought intrusion, and avoidance are all based on memory of the traumatic event, while amnesia for the event can be a component of TBI. Put more simply: how can one suffer flashbacks for events one cannot remember? Or, how can one avoid something one cannot remember? As convincing as this logic might seem, most clinicians believe TBI and PTSD can co-exist, especially in active duty service members and veterans. The argument against the coexistence of PTSD and TBI is inherently flawed when applied to the combat setting. It is quite possible for soldiers to experience a TBI, but also have PTSD from other events experienced (not the TBI-causing event) during their deployment. In addition, many of the service members serving in OEF/OIF have sustained a mild TBI, where a loss of consciousness and amnesia for the event are not necessary conditions. Indeed, researchers found that 25% of veterans with TBI also met criteria for PTSD.[25] Other estimates of the prevalence of PTSD among active duty OEF/OIF service members and veterans range from 12% to 24%.[26–28] Several of the symptoms of PTSD overlap with those seen following a TBI, thus complicating the clinical picture.

TREATMENT

The primary goals for treating TBI and PTSD include reducing symptoms, relieving comorbid symptoms, improving functioning, and strengthening resilience.[29,30]

All treatment approaches described in this section propose to accomplish these four goals. Reduction of TBI symptoms and relief of comorbid symptoms (eg, anxiety, depression, and PTSD) are directly addressed, and in doing so, everyday functioning improves. The pharmacologic treatments commonly employed by nurses are described. The treatments discussed have been proven to be beneficial to those with TBI, but may not have been studied directly in the active duty military or veteran population. It is also important to note that some of the medications recommended may not be included in the VA formulary thus may be inappropriate in the VA setting.

It is not clear whether the cognitive and behavioral deficits found in TBI adversely affect pharmacologic treatment.[31] Pharmacotherapy of TBI presents a challenge, because the very nature of TBIs indicates an alteration in brain function. Because of this, a dimension to drug response is added that may not occur in the general population or in other individuals requiring psychotropic medications. While one veteran might respond in an expected manner, another might respond in a very unique way. TBI patients can be overly sensitive to psychotropic medications, again related to the brain injury, or can be unusually drug-resistant.[29,32] Of course, this creates a prescribing dilemma for clinicians: being alert for the hypersensitive patient while not undertreating the drug-resistant patient. Because of this variance in sensitivity, it is important to start low and go slow.[33] Potentially this creates the possibility of lengthening the process of finding the right drug at the right dosage, thus making the process tedious for both patient and clinician.[34]

Typically treatment is symptom-based: antidepressants for depression, antipsychotics for psychosis, mood stabilizers for mood swings and irritability, anxiolytics for anxiety, and cognitive enhancers for cognitive problems.

Depression is the most common psychiatric sequela of TBI.[35] It is appropriate to follow traditional approaches for depression within the veteran population. For example, TBI-induced depression can be treated with sertraline (50–200 mg/d), paroxetine (20–60 mg/d), citalopram (20–60 mg/d), and other selective serotonin reuptake inhibitors (SSRIs) with positive results. Some patients may be ordered a tricyclic antidepressant such as amitriptyline (up to 300 mg/d) and desipramine (150–300 mg/d). A guiding principle for pharmacotherapy is the minimization of anticholinergic and sedative effects while not lowering the seizure threshold.[36] The latter emphasis is particularly significant for a population who might be more vulnerable to seizures because of their TBI. Anxiety is almost as common among these individuals as depression.[35] Most often, anxiety is treated with a short-term benzodiazepine such as lorazepam or perhaps alprazolam, while simultaneously prescribing an SSRI. Short-term use of the benzodiazepines is purposeful because of the addictive nature of these drugs. The emerging evidence of a link between TBI and substance abuse[37] warrants further elucidation of this potential association. In the meantime, prudence dictates that benzodiazepines be used as stabilizing medications until the SSRIs take effect. An effective teaching point for the veteran (and all patients being treated with these drugs for anxiety) is to compare the benzodiazepines to aspirin and the SSRIs to an anti-biotic. The aspirin (ie, the lorazepam) has an immediate effect but only addresses symp-toms (ie, as soon as the aspirin wears off the pain returns). The antibiotic (ie, the SSRI) treats the underlying problem (ie, kills the bug). Hopefully, the patient will stabilize within a few weeks and treatment with benzodiazepine can be eliminated from the regimen.

Manic symptoms are thankfully rare.[23,24] If they do develop, traditional dosages of divalproex or lithium are recommended.[36] Common dosages for divalproex (up to 60 mg/kg/d) and serum levels (85–125 μg/mL) should be observed. Lithium serum level parameters (0.6–1.2 mEq/L) remain important for this population and since lithium is known to cause cognitive dulling and lower seizure thresholds, many clinicians use it only if divalproex is ineffective.

Psychosis is also a relatively unlikely sequela of TBI.[25] Atypical antipsychotics are most likely to be prescribed should hallucinatory or delusional thinking develop. Olan-zapine (5–20 mg/d) and quetiapine (300–800 mg/d) can be used.[38]

As noted, cognitive symptoms are relatively common disabilities associated with TBIs. While cognitive–behavioral therapy is the recommended treatment of choice for PTSD by the Institutes of Medicine, cognitive changes may render it less effective in the treatment of TBI. The very nature of this therapy is heavily reliant on memory, which may be compromised as a result of the TBI. This reality may make pharmacotherapy for cognitive symptoms even more significant. Since the ability to attend and a decrease in alertness are core problems, methylphenidate is recommended at a dose range of 0.25 to 0.30 mg/kg twice per day. It is also effective for the reduced speed of mental process-ing, about which many of these veterans complain.[32,38] Donepezil (5–10 mg/d) is occa-sionally prescribed for attention deficits.[32] Other medications that may prove effective in reducing TBI cognitive symptoms include modafinil and atomoxetine.

Finally, and perhaps of most concern to patients, families, and clinicians, are the aggressive symptoms that can occur in TBI patients. Because aggressive behaviors raise safety risks and since these behaviors frighten others, it is important for the patient, the family, and the nurse to deal with them quickly.[34] Pharmacotherapy includes beta-blockers for potentially problematic behaviors. Propranolol (up to 520 mg/d) and pindolol (up to 100 mg/d) have been used effectively.[36] Methylphenidate also has proven a surprisingly effective tool for agitation.[33,38] Other medications proven effective for aggression include divalproex, lithium, SSRIs (particularly sertraline and paroxetine), tricyclic antidepressants, and buspirone (10–60 mg/d).[36] Again, since aggressive behaviors are frightening to those around the veteran, the behaviors must be addressed quickly. It is important to listen to both the patient's and the family's concerns, as family members are often an important ally in the treatment regimen.[39]

CASE STUDIES
Case 1, Severe TBI

Veteran A is a young man who served two tours in Iraq as a Marine. He sustained an injury while in Iraq due to a bullet from a sniper, which penetrated his skull in the left temporal region. The details of the injury are unclear, but it was estimated that he had a 10-day loss of consciousness. He had a GCS score of 6 upon admission to the hospital. The head computed tomography (CT) scan showed a large left temporal skull fracture, fragments to the brain midline, and extensive hemorrhaging with laceration to the left middle cerebral artery. Blood was present in the lateral and third ventricles, and hydrocephalus was evident. When his condition stabilized, he underwent surgical repair for his head injury. Recovery from the acute episode of the trauma required several months, after which he was admitted to the rehabilitation unit. Postinjury disability included right hemiplegia, nonfluent aphasia, and right visual field deficit. Following inpatient rehabilitation, he was discharged home. He continued to receive outpatient therapy focusing on language skills while participating in regular physical exercise to increase strength and balance.

Several years after injury, he had made improvements, but continued to evidence diminished expressive and receptive language skills, a right visual field deficit, and a dense right upper extremity paresis. His language abilities made it difficult to obtain a clear picture of his true emotional functioning, but he did manifest symptoms of PTSD (nightmares, flashbacks, hypervigilance, and hyperarousal) that improved over a period of several years. Although he expressed feelings of frustration due to his limitations, his mood was generally good. Veteran A remains active by participating in hobbies and playing on the computer.

Case 2, Mild TBI

As is typical in those who have experienced a mild, combat-related TBI, there were no records or documentation of the injury that caused the trauma. In the case of Veteran B, he reported two injuries sustained during service in Iraq but records of the injuries were not available. The first occurred when the vehicle in which he was traveling hit a landmine. Per the veteran's report, he hit his head on the ceiling of the vehicle, but did not experience any loss or change in consciousness. He denied any PTA or postconcussive symptoms after that event. Several months later, he was traveling in a vehicle and was exposed to an IED blast approximately 2 meters from his position. Veteran B reportedly was "tossed around" inside of the vehicle and had a brief loss of consciousness lasting seconds, but he denied PTA. Rather, he reported a headache and tightness in his chest after that event. He did not seek treatment after either of the incidents, continued to perform his duties following the injuries, and completed his tour with no difficulty.

He presented for care at the VA several years later, with numerous physical, cognitive, and emotional complaints. He reported chronic headaches, insomnia, tinnitus, and chronic pain as well as difficulty with cognitive skills, including attention, concentration, and word finding. Finally, he reported symptoms consistent with PTSD. Veteran B was able to maintain employment despite these numerous symptoms. He received regular mental health treatment through the VA. He completed cognitive processing therapy (CPT), which is an evidence-based treatment for PTSD that focuses on education about PTSD, the relationship between thoughts and feelings, processing of the trauma, challenging of thoughts regarding the event, and finally, restructuring of the thoughts regarding the traumatic event.

CONCLUDING THOUGHTS

Since September 2001, over 1.6 million service members have served in combat situations in Iraq or Afghanistan.[1] As of June 2010, there were 92,000 service members in Iraq, and an additional 94,000 service members were based in Afghanistan. Of these, tens of thousands have been spared death through improved body armor and emergency care, but have sustained injuries such as TBIs. While numbers on a piece of paper quickly lose potency, the message gleaned from these statistics should be the awareness that families, health care agencies, and society can expect to see more and not less of the injuries described in this article. Long-term effects on the service member are yet to be understood. In the meantime, it behooves those who work with and care for these service members and veterans to be aware of TBIs, be knowledgeable about TBI care, and be supportive of those who have sacrificed their health and well-being for others.

REFERENCES

1. Tanielian T, Jaycox LH, Schell T, et al. Invisible wounds of war: summary and recommendations for addressing psychological and cognitive injuries. Santa Monica (CA): Rand Corporation; 2008.
2. Warden D. Military TBI during the Iraq and Afghanistan wars. J Head Trauma Rehabil 2006;21:398–402.
3. Schwab KA, Warden D, Lux WE, et al. Defense and veterans brain injury center: peacetime and wartime missions. J Rehabil Res Dev 2007;44(7):xiii–xxi.
4. Okie S. Reconstructing lives—a tale of two soldiers. N Engl J Med 2006;355: 2609–15.
5. Parker RS. Concussive brain trauma. Neurobehavioral impairment and maladaptation. Boca Raton (FL): CRC Press; 2001.
6. Richardson JTE. Clinical and neuropsychological aspects of closed head injury. 2nd edition. London: Taylor & Francis; 2000.
7. McCrea MA. Mild traumatic brain injury and postconcussion syndrome: the new evidence base for diagnosis and treatment. Oxford (UK): Oxford University Press; 2008.
8. Teasdale G, Jennett B. Assessment of coma and impaired consciousness: a practical scale. Lancet 1974;2(7872):81–4.
9. Fischer JS, Hannay J, Loring DW, et al. Observational methods, rating scales, and inventories. In: Lezak MD, Howieson DB, Loring DW, editors. Neuropsychological assessment. 4th edition. Oxford (UK): Oxford University Press; 2004.
10. Stuss DT, Binns MA, Carruth FG, et al. The acute period of recovery from traumatic brain injury: post-traumatic amnesia or posttraumatic confusional state? J Neurosurg 1999;90:635–43.
11. Bishara SN, Partridge FM, Godfrey HP, et al. Post-traumatic amnesia and Glasgow Coma Scale related to outcome in survivors in a consecutive series of patients with severe closed-head injury. Brain Inj 1992;6:373–80.
12. DePalma RG, Burris DG, Champion HR, et al. Blast injuries. N Engl J Med 2005; 352(13):1335–42.
13. Hoge CW, McGurk D, Thomas JL, et al. Mild traumatic brain injury in U.S. soldiers returning from Iraq. N Engl J Med 2008;358:453–63.
14. Stein MB, Mcallister TW. Exploring the convergence of posttraumatic stress disorder and mild traumatic brain injury. Am J Psychiatry 2009;166:768–76.
15. Hugenholtz H, Stuss DT, Stethem LL, et al. How long does it take to recover from a mild concussion? Neurosurgery 1988;22:853–8.
16. Sohlberg MM, Mateer CA. Cognitive rehabilitation: an integrative neuropsychological approach. 2nd edition. New York: Taylor & Guilford Press; 2001.

17. Bate AJ, Mathias JL, Crawford JR. Performance on the test of everyday attention and standard tests of attention following severe traumatic brain injury. Clin Neuropsychol 2001;15:405–22.
18. Zec RF, Zellers D, Belman J, et al. Long-term consequences of severe closed head injury on episodic memory. J Clin Exp Neuropsychol 2001;23:671–91.
19. Swaine BR, Sullivan SJ. Longitudinal profile of early motor recovery following severe traumatic brain injury. Brain Inj 1996;10:347–66.
20. Crosson B, Barco PP, Velozo CA, et al. Awareness and compensation in postacute head injury rehabilitation. J Head Trauma Rehabil 1989;4:46–54.
21. Jorge RE, Robinson RG, Arndt SV, et al. Comparison between acute- and delayed-onset depression following traumatic brain injury. J Neuropsychiatry Clin Neurosci 1993;5(1):43–9.
22. Gomez-Hernandez R, Max JE, Kosier T, et al. Social impairment and depression after traumatic brain injury. Arch Phys Med Rehabil 1997;78:1321–6.
23. Jorge RE, Robinson RG, Starkstein SE, et al. Secondary mania following traumatic brain injury. Am J Psychiatry 1993;150:916–21.
24. Van Reekum R, Cohen T, Wong J. Can traumatic brain injury cause psychiatric disorders? J Neuropsychiatry Clin Neurosci 2000;12:316–27.
25. Kim E, Lauterbach EC, Reeve A, et al. Neuropsychiatric complications of traumatic brain injury: a critical review of the literature (a report of the ANPA Committee on Research). J Neuropsychiatry Clin Neurosci 2007;19(2):106–27.
26. Milliken CS, Auchterlonie JL, Hoge CW. Longitudinal assessment of mental health problems among active and reserve component soldiers returning from the Iraq War. JAMA 2007;298:2141–8.
27. Seal KH, Metzler TJ, Gima KS, et al. Trends and risk factors for mental health diagnoses among Iraq and Afghanistan veterans using Department of Veterans Affairs health care, 2002–2008. Am J Public Health 2009;99:1651–8.
28. Seal KH, Berthenthal D, Miner CR, et al. Bringing the war back home: mental health disorders among 103,788 US veterans returning from Iraq and Afghanistan seen at Department of Veterans Affairs facilities. Arch Intern Med 2007;167:476–82.
29. Davidson JR. Pharmacologic treatment of acute and chronic stress following trauma. J Clin Psychiatry 2006;67(Suppl 2):34–9.
30. Dowben JS, Grant JS, Keltner NL. Psychobiological substrates of posttraumatic stress disorder: part II. Perspect Psychiatr Care 2007;43(3):146–9.
31. Vasterling JJ, Verfaellie M, Sullivan KD. Mild traumatic brain injury and posttraumatic stress disorder in returning veterans: perspectives from cognitive neuroscience. Clin Psychol Rev 2009;29:674–84.
32. Tenovuo O. Pharmacological enhancement of cognitive and behavioral decifits after traumatic brain injury. Trauma Rehabil 2006;52:2–11.
33. Ashman T, Gordon W, Cantor J, et al. Neurobehavioral consequences of traumatic brain injury. Mt Sinai J Med 2006;73:999–1005.
34. Keltner NL, McGuinness JP. War related psychiatric disorders in soldiers. In: Keltner NL, Bostrom C, McGuinness T, editors. Psychiatric nursing. 6th edition. St Louis (MO): Elsevier; 2011. p. 489–98.
35. Martin EM, Lu WC, Helmick K, et al. Traumatic brain injuries sustained in the Afghanistan and Iraq wars. Am J Nurs 2008;108(4):40–7.
36. Cooke BB, Keltner NL. Traumatic brain injury-war related: part II. Perspect Psychiatr Care 2008;44(1):54–7.
37. Whelan-Goodinson R, Ponsford J, Johnston L, et al. Psychiatric disorders following traumatic brain injury: their nature and frequency. J Head Trauma Rehabil 2009;24:324–32.

38. Neurobehavioral Guidelines Working Group, Warden DL, Gordon B, et al. Guidelines for the pharmacologic treatment of neurobehavioral sequelae of traumatic brain injury. J Neurotrauma 2006;23:1468–501.
39. Anderson MI, Simpson GK, Morey PJ, et al. Differential pathways of psychological distress in spouses vs. parents of people with severe traumatic brain injury (TBI): multi-group analysis. Brain Inj 2009;23:931–43.

Substance Abuse Interface with Intimate Partner Violence: What Treatment Programs Need to Know

Margaret H. Brackley, PhD, RN[a,b,*], Gail B. Williams, PhD, RN[a,b], Christina C. Wei, PhD, RN[a]

KEYWORDS

- Intimate partner violence • Substance abuse
- Treatment protocols

On national surveys, intimate partner violence (IPV) is estimated to affect between 12% and 14% of women annually.[1] Substance abuse (SA) in either partner increases the risk of family violence. About 44% of men entering alcohol treatment programs have self-reported being violent toward their partners within the pretreatment year.[1] Because SA treatment programs are potentially an important entry into treatment for men who abuse their partners, such programs have been encouraged to screen for IPV. In 1997, the Substance Abuse and Mental Health Services Administration issued the Treatment Improvement Protocol Series (TIPS) number 25: *Substance Abuse Treatment and Domestic Violence* to provide consensus on how treatment programs should respond to IPV.[2] Reported surveys indicate that few programs have the suggested processes and procedures in place to screen and intervene with survivors and perpetrators of IPV.[3]

DEFINITION

According to the Centers for Disease Control and Prevention, there is value in a common scientific definition of a study phenomenon.[4] There is a general consensus in the violence prevention scientific community to use the term intimate partner

[a] Department of Family and Community Health Systems, The University of Texas Health Science Center at San Antonio, 7703 Floyd Curl Drive, San Antonio, TX 78229-3900, USA
[b] Center for Violence Prevention, San Antonio, TX, USA
* Corresponding author. Department of Family and Community Health Systems, The University of Texas Health Science Center at San Antonio, 7703 Floyd Curl Drive, San Antonio, TX 78229-3900.
E-mail address: brackley@uthscsa.edu

Nurs Clin N Am 45 (2010) 581–589
doi:10.1016/j.cnur.2010.06.001
0029-6465/10/$ – see front matter © 2010 Elsevier Inc. All rights reserved.
nursing.theclinics.com

violence to describe physical, sexual, or psychological harm by a current or former intimate partner or spouse. This type of violence can occur among heterosexual or same-sex couples and does not require sexual intimacy. TIPS number 25 focuses on men who abuse their female partners, but concepts could be extended to same-sex relationships as well.

PREVALENCE OF IPV

Each year, women experience about 4.8 million intimate partner–related physical assaults and rapes.[5] Most police-reported survivors of IPV are women and most IPV offenders are men. Between 2001 and 2005, nonfatal IPV against women made up 22% of all nonfatal violence victimizations against girls aged 12 years or older and 4% of nonfatal violence victimizations against boys aged 12 years or older.[1] About 11% of all murders were by intimates, but one-third of women were murdered by an intimate partner.[1] Approximately 96% of women who experienced nonfatal IPV reported that they were victimized by a man, whereas approximately 82% of men who experienced nonfatal IPV reported that they were victimized by a woman.[1] Women aged 35 to 49 years and those who are separated, divorced, or never married may be at the greatest risk for IPV.[1] However, non–police-reported incidents of IPV have found that IPV perpetration may occur more equally between women and men (consider this substitution for the sexes). Findings from a 2002 meta-analysis by Archer[6] found an equal prevalence of IPV between genders. The most frequent reason for not reporting IPV to the police was that the incident was a private or personal matter.[1]

PREVALENCE OF CO-OCCURRENCE OF IPV AND SA

On average, between 2001 and 2005, the use of any alcohol or drugs was reported by IPV survivors in about 42% of all nonfatal IPV incidents reported to the police.[1] With regard to the interface of IPV and SA, findings reveal that the odds of any male-to-female violence for those who relapsed to alcohol use were more than 3.7 times higher than for those who did not.[7] In addition, among those who relapsed to alcohol use, the odds of male-to-female severe violence were almost 6 times greater than those who did not.[7] This finding is consistent with the literature, because studies in this area have reliably revealed that roughly 50% of married or cohabiting patients entering treatment for SA reported one or more episodes of partner violence in the year preceding treatment.[8]

PREVENTION OF INJURY

For the period 2001 to 2005, on average, less than one-fifth of survivors of nonfatal IPV who reported an injury sought treatment after the injury.[1] In addition, for the same period, half of all women who experienced nonfatal IPV suffered an injury from their victimization; about 5% were seriously injured and about 44% suffered minor injuries.[1] For men during the same period, on average, more than one-third of IPV survivors were injured; 4% were seriously injured and 36% suffered minor injuries.[1]

MISSED OPPORTUNITY: FAILURE TO IDENTIFY IPV

Failure to identify survivors of IPV can lead to risks for homicide, exposure of dependent children to IPV, and mental illness. Schumacher and colleagues[9] found that 44% of the men who entered 7 treatment programs self-reported at least one act of IPV in the pretreatment year. On examination of the treatment record, only 17% of these men had been screened and referred for IPV treatment. The investigators relate that 83% of the men were either not screened or the screening method used was ineffective or referrals were not given. Campbell and colleagues[10] report that there are missed opportunities and increased risk factors for homicide when health care providers do not identify IPV. Failure to identify child survivors of IPV may lead to the intergenerational transmission of IPV. On average, between 2001 and 2005, in households experiencing IPV, children were present in 38% of the violent incidents involving female survivors and in 21% of the incidents involving male victims.[1] Moreover, the literature suggests that having experienced violence as a child is a risk factor for later perpetration of IPV and SA.[11]

Results of a bivariate analysis indicated that adults with a history of IPV and childhood abuse report greater disruptions in their self-appraisals and a greater likelihood of mental and SA disorders than adults with no IPV experience.[12] Specifically, those who experienced IPV were more dependent on and more enmeshed with others, felt more insecure, and had lower self-esteem. These adults were also more likely to have depression, anxiety, posttraumatic stress disorder symptoms, and alcohol and SA problems.

SCREENING

The US Preventive Services Task Force (USPSTF) found insufficient evidence to recommend for or against routine screening for IPV in women.[13] However, the USPSTF stated that no studies have directly addressed the harms of screening and interventions for IPV, and as a result, the USPSTF could not determine the balance between the benefits and harms of screening for IPV among women. According to the USPSTF, women screened for IPV reported no harmful effects of screening.[13] In addition, the USPSTF reported that there were no existing studies that determined the accuracy of screening tools used to identify IPV in women. Although there is insufficient evidence to evaluate whether screening effectively reduces violence against women or associated negative outcomes, health care settings may provide a unique confidential opportunity for survivors of IPV to seek help. Despite a lack of confirmed efficacy, routine screening of women for IPV is still strongly recommended by panels of experts on IPV.[14] On the other hand, no clinical recommendations exist for routine screening of perpetrators and male survivors of IPV.

Safety

Safety must be the foundation of any intervention for IPV. Treatment providers who lack knowledge, skills, and appropriate attitudes related to IPV screening can unintentionally cause harm. For example, the most dangerous time for families that have experienced violence is when a partner leaves. Furthermore, this practice has been shown to put women and children at risk for injury and even death.[10] Therefore, a health care provider or staff who encourages an abused woman to leave her situation without a plan to ensure her safety contributes to risk.

Much of what is known by researching cases of death and near death of women is counterintuitive to common thought. For example, informing the abusive partner about the intention to leave seems to be good communication, but most women are killed or injured in response to the abusive partner's new awareness that she is leaving. Developing a safety plan is essential to providing quality evidence-based care for abused women.[10]

Skills and Tools

Examples of skills and tools needed to provide best practices for clients experiencing both IPV and SA included in TIPS 25[2] are

- Two-minute screening for domestic violence and brief intervention
- Conducting a danger assessment for lethality

- Safety planning
- Assessing conflict within couples
- Intervention to gain survivor's trust
- Compliance strategies for SA treatment
- Community resource development.

The examples of the recommended screening tools and interventions are included in TIPS 25 and can be retrieved at http://www.ncbi.nlm.nih.gov/bookshelf/br.fcgi?book=hssamhsatip.

Two-minute screen for domestic violence and brief intervention

Couples entering treatment need to be screened individually and privately. Agencies need to establish procedures to ensure time for private screening, which takes approximately 2 minutes if negative and an additional 8 minutes if positive. It is feasible to perform IPV screening while urine samples are being obtained or paperwork is being completed. It is best practice to make IPV screening a standard procedure so that everyone becomes familiar with being separated during the admission process. If a partner is not accompanying the significant other to the treatment facility, IPV screening could be done over the phone when the patient is in the treatment facility thus ensuring privacy. If the results of the IPV screen are negative, it is best to inform the person that sometimes this changes during treatment and if it does, help is available. If the results of the IPV screen are positive, then a danger assessment and safety plan should be completed. If danger is found to be imminent or high, then the police or an IPV shelter can be called. People experiencing abuse should be informed that no one deserves abuse and that it is not their fault. Resources/referrals should be given and safety plans completed. Training of staff to complete this brief intervention is needed because even providing a brochure to a survivor in an abusive relationship can increase their risk of injury should the abuser find the brochure.

Screening of persons who may inflict violence can be accomplished by asking direct questions such as "In my practice, I find some patients with similar situations to yours will on occasion yell, threaten, or hit their partners or other family members. Has this happened to you?" Educate patients that even if the person is not seriously hurt, there can be long-lasting problems for children and partners after experiencing this behavior. Also, they need to be told that it is a crime to threaten or hit someone even if it is a family member. Intervention can be done by offering referrals to violence prevention programs that can be found by calling the national hotline number.

Conducting a danger assessment for lethality

SA treatment is generally recognized as a family intervention. Family members may have insisted on entering the treatment. Failure to identify violence in the family can interfere with treatment and contribute to relapse. Families are encouraged to engage in treatment activities because they are an important source of support in posttreatment sobriety. Couples therapy is often a component of SA treatment. Violence in couples in therapy is underreported and often not identified unless specifically addressed. Couples therapy is based on the assumption of equality within the dyad. Equality is not possible if IPV is a factor in a relationship. Therefore, couples therapy has not been recommended for couples with IPV, citing it as potentially dangerous and even unethical. Recent research, however, has challenged this notion and has shown that couples therapy under certain circumstances may be an effective treatment for partners experiencing both IPV and SA.[1]

In several studies, "couples-based treatment designed to address alcohol use and relationship problems led to greater reductions in IPV than alcoholism treatment only."[15] There are recommendations related to the level of violence and current abstinence from substances related to which couples are appropriate for this kind of treatment. Couples who are not candidates are those in which one or both partners report (1) fear of injury, death, or physical reprisal from their partner; (2) severe violence requiring hospitalization within the last 2 years; (3) threat of harm to either with a weapon; (4) fear of participating in couples therapy; or (5) wanting to leave the relationship because of partners' severity of aggression.[16] Whether couples therapy is used or not, safety planning is essential to providing evidence-based intervention.

Safety planning

Personalized safety plans are included in comprehensive materials developed for TIPS 25. The plans are easy to understand and to explain to women and children. Safety is important for all members of a violent family. Safety is particularly important as treatment progresses when working with couples. A completed safety plan should be included in the medical record. Safety plans have shown to be an effective way to prevent violence and resulting injuries in families.

Assessing conflict within couples

The Conflict Tactics Scale (CTS) is a widely used and recognized tool that measures the extent to which partners in dating, cohabiting, or marital relationships engage in psychological and physical attacks on each other. The scale also measures their use of reasoning or negotiation to deal with conflicts. Use of the CTS facilitates identification of partners experiencing physical, psychological, and sexual abuse as well as physical injury related to the violence. Since 1972, the CTS has been used in numerous studies in at least 20 countries involving more than 70,000 informants from diverse cultural backgrounds. In 1994, articles that reported findings based on the CTS were published at a rate of approximately 10 per month. The revised CTS2 has a new format that simplifies administration and reduces response set and requires only a sixth grade reading ability.[17] Reported reliability for the CTS2 ranges from 0.79 to 0.95.[17] Because the CTS2 contains physical, psychological, and sexual abuse scales, it fosters a more conceptualized and comprehensive assessment of abuse/violence in relationships than other instruments. Assessment using CTS2 takes approximately 15 minutes.

The revised CTS2 is a 78-item tool consisting of 5 subscales (negotiation, psychological aggression, physical assault, sexual coercion, and injury). By means of the subscales, these 5 types of conflict tactics or violence can be measured. The CTS2 also measures prevalence of IPV in terms of prevalence, chronicity, annual frequency, and ever prevalence. The psychological aggression, physical assault, sexual coercion, and injury scales are further divided into minor and severe acts. Although there is no composite score for the CTS2, the subscale scores provide a rich description of the types of conflict tactics or violence that partners engage in and valuable information about the prevalence, chronicity, and annual frequency of such violence. Additional information and instrument items are listed in TIPS 25.

Interventions to gain the survivor's trust

All screening and intervention should occur within the context of a therapeutic relationship. Basic trust building is the foundation of a therapeutic relationship. Everyone working in SA treatment programs should aim to be consistent, reliable, and trustworthy with patients. Abused persons are highly sensitive and sometimes hypervigilant to their environments. It is useful to remember that both parties in a violent relationship may have histories of childhood abuse and childhood witnessing of IPV. Trust becomes even more important for these patients.

Community resource development

A community assessment of services available to survivors and perpetrators of IPV is ideal. Once identified, agencies can make agreements with both the police and the Battered Women's Shelter services for immediate dangers and referral. Many police and sheriff departments have specialized training and personnel in place to handle IPV. In more remote rural areas, there may be a reluctance to call either, fearing that confidentiality will be breached. The national hotline number is available to give information on what to do and how to do. Often communities transport persons needing a safe haven to another community for services.

There is some evidence that providing colocated or integrated IPV and SA services in the same site are beneficial to women with SA problems. If these services are not available, then it is important to get to know one's community so that there are ready sources and agreements with referrals to community, private, and public resources. Safety planning training is needed for personnel so that many different staff can provide this essential service. Women have special issues to face if they have children. There are few treatment programs that have child care services in many areas of the country. If the woman needs inpatient treatment, housing must include children or else the mother may lose custody of her children.

Compliance strategies

Gender-specific treatment programs for IPV are desirable because men and women face different problems due to SA and IPV. Mandatory reporting of IPV is not indicated unless the survivor is younger than 18 years or older than 65 years, is disabled, or was attacked by a weapon that requires reporting in most states. In states where mandatory reporting occurs for medical professionals, lay screeners may be used to avoid reporting, if the client wants the provider not to report. Mandatory reporting may facilitate data collection and the persecution of perpetrators but violates the ethical code of nursing, which calls for supporting the autonomy and rights of patients. It may put the survivor at risk for more abuse, and there is no way to guarantee that the survivor will be protected from harm as evidenced by the number of deaths of women who had protective court orders for abusers.

When indicated, male perpetrators of IPV may be referred to mental health services. Although male perpetrators mandated to mental health services showed no decrease in violence, men who participated in mental health treatment showed a decrease in violence toward their partners.[12] Hence, male perpetrators with mental health problems should be referred to mental health services.

Barriers to Implementation of TIPS 25

Staff may not feel prepared to deal with IPV.[18] Regardless of the intervention used, some couples may remain violent. Staff may become involved and with involvement comes the risk of vicarious traumatization. Without training, staff may offer advice that puts the person at a greater-than-ordinary risk or isolates the person further. Therefore, staff must have training to offset potential of statements that may put the survivor of IPV at risk. Types of statements to avoid violence include "tell him you are leaving if he doesn't stop" and "I would not put up with this, I respect myself more." Potential outcomes of statements like these may put the IPV survivor in increased danger, because if survivors follow the former statement and believe that they are not worthy, they may decide to quit telling people about the abuse. In addition, anything that seems to take time away from treatment increases resistance and anxiety in staff.

Suggested Ways to Make it Work

Agencies can provide widespread training so that many types of staff, from receptionists to providers, can screen, do safety planning, and provide referral materials. Many times, it is the office receptionist, and not the providers, who is the first to hear about abuse. Placing materials in the waiting areas about common triggers of abuse can encourage clients to talk to staff about abuse. Posters, brochures, and materials about healthy relationships that are distributed during assessments or placed in the waiting room can bring attention to the issue of IPV. Materials from referral sources such as National Hotline for Domestic Violence (1-800-799-SAFE [7233]) can also be useful.

WHAT ROLE DO NURSES PLAY IN IPV/SA SCREENING, INTERVENTION, AND REFERRAL?

The generalist nurse needs to learn to screen for IPV and to know how to help if the screening result is positive. **Table 1** provides the knowledge, skills, and attitudes needed by the nurse for this type of screening, intervention, and referral.

Advanced Practice Nurses

Advanced practice nurses (APNs)/nurses with Doctorate in Nursing Practice (DNP) who are involved in IPV or SA treatment should learn to integrate care and improve processes for ensuring the safety of clients and their partners and the quality of care that they receive. The APNs/nurses with DNP can provide value to an agency by developing gender-specific interventions as well as services for children related with IPV and SA. Prevention foci aimed at ameliorating the long-term effects of growing up in a home where IPV and SA are practiced can stop the intergenerational transmission of both IPV and SA.

Table 1
Summary of knowledge, skills, and attitudes needed by the generalist nurse for IPV screening

Knowledge	Skills	Attitudes
Strategies that promote safety while implementing a caring nurse-patient relationship for both individuals in a violent relationship	How to assess and respond appropriately to the level of risk involved in experiences of depression, suicide, psychosis, aggression (violence), and SA across the life span and clinical encounters/sites of care	Empathy and unconditional regard for persons who live with violence plus a nonjudgmental attitude
The best practices that promote safety and create a just and safe environment for both partners	How to evaluate a client's living situation for safety, structure, and support	Intellectual curiosity and cultural awareness about best practices and individual living variations plus a value for social justice
	How to promote safety with correct reporting and interventions if the patient becomes violent toward the partner or self	Concern for safety and understanding about the need to take action

Treatment issues at the interface of IPV and SA are numerous. Nursing can play an important role despite the nurse being in practice at the generalist or advanced level. Learning the skills for intervening with these complex patients and their families adds to the nurse's ability to prevent both SA and IPV in the next generation.

REFERENCES

1. Catalano S. Intimate partner violence in the United States. 2007. Available at: http://www.ojp.usdoj.gov/bjs/intimate/ipv.htm. Accessed December 1, 2009.
2. Center for Substance Abuse Treatment. Substance abuse and domestic violence. Treatment improvement protocol (TIP) series, No. 25. DHHS Publication No. (SMA) 97-3163. Rockville (MD): Substance Abuse and Mental Health Services Administration; 1997. Available at: http://www.ncbi.nlm.nih.gov/bookshelf/br.fcgi?book=hssamhsatip&part=A46712. Accessed November 10, 2009.
3. Bennett LW. Substance abuse by men in partner abuse intervention programs: current issues and promising trends. Violence Vict 2008;23:236–48.
4. Saltzman LE, Fanslow JL, McMahon PM, et al. Intimate partner violence surveillance: uniform definitions and recommended data elements, version 1.0. Atlanta (GA): Centers for Disease Control and Prevention, National Center for Injury Prevention and Control; 2002. Available at: http://www.cdc.gov/ncipc/pub-res/ipv_surveillance/intimate.htm. Accessed July 19, 2010.
5. Tjaden P, Thoennes N. Extent, nature, and consequences of intimate partner violence: findings from the national Violence Against Women Survey. Publication No. NCJ 181867. Washington, DC: Department of Justice (US); 2000. Available at: www.ojp.usdoj.gov/nij/pubs-sum/181867.htm. Accessed July 19, 2010.
6. Archer JC. Sex differences in aggression between heterosexual partners: a meta-analytic review. Psychol Bull 2000;126(5):651–80.
7. Mignone T, Klostermann K, Chen R. The relationship between relapse to alcohol and relapse to violence. J Fam Violence 2009;24(7):497–505.
8. Fals-Stewart W, Clinton-Sherrod M. Treating intimate partner violence among substance-abusing dyads: the effect of couples therapy. Prof Psychol Res Pract 2009;40(3):257–63.
9. Schumacher JA, Fals-Stewart W, Leonard KE. Domestic violence treatment referrals for men seeking alcohol treatment. J Subst Abuse Treat 2003;24(3):279–83.
10. Campbell JC, Webster D, Koziol-McLain J, et al. Assessing risk factors for intimate partner homicide. NIJ J 2003;250:14–9 Available at: http://ncjrs.org/pdffiles1/jr000250e.pdf. Accessed July 19, 2010.
11. Gil-Gonzalez D, Vives-Cases C, Ruiz MT, et al. Childhood experiences of violence in perpetrators as a risk factor of intimate partner violence: a systematic review. J Publ Health 2007;30(1):14–22.
12. Gondolf EW. Outcomes from referring batterer program participants to mental health treatment. J Fam Violence 2009;24(8):577–88.
13. U.S. Preventive Services Task Force. Screening for family and intimate partner violence. Ann Intern Med 2004;140:382–6.
14. Family Violence Prevention Fund, Inc. The National Consensus Guidelines on identifying and responding to domestic violence victimization in health care settings. Available at: http://www.endabuse.org/programs/healthcare/files/Consensus.pdf. Accessed November 10, 2009.
15. Powers MB, Vedel E, Emmelkamp PM. Behavioral couples therapy (BCT) for alcohol and drug use disorders: a meta-analysis. Clin Psychol Rev 2008;28(6):952–62.

16. Fals-Stewart W, Kennedy C. Addressing intimate partner violence in substance abuse treatment: overview, options, and recommendations. J Subst Abuse Treat 2005;29:5–17.
17. Straus M, Hamby S, Boney-McCoy S, et al. The revised conflict tactics scales (CTS2): development and preliminary psychometric data. J Fam Issues 1996; 17(3):283–316.
18. Kunins H, Gilbert L, Whyte-Etere A, et al. Substance abuse treatment staff perceptions of intimate partner victimization among female clients. J Psychoactive Drugs 2007;39(3):251–7.

Medical Illnesses in People with Schizophrenia

Peggy El-Mallakh, PhD, RN[a,*], Patricia B. Howard, PhD, RN, CNAA, FAAN[a],
Brittany N. Evans, BA, BSN, RN[b]

KEYWORDS

- Schizophrenia • Medical illnesses • Access to care
- Psychiatric nursing

Mental health clinicians and researchers are increasingly focused on the epidemiology, cause, and treatment of physical illnesses of people with schizophrenia. A growing body of research indicates that approximately 50% to 60% of people with schizophrenia have at least 1 comorbid chronic medical illness[1,2]; up to 83% of those with co-occurring schizophrenia and alcohol dependence have at least 1 comorbid medical illness.[3] Furthermore, chronic illnesses such as hypertension, diabetes, and metabolic syndrome are more prevalent among those with schizophrenia compared with the general population.[1,4–6]

High rates of chronic illnesses among those with schizophrenia are associated with high mortality and reduced life expectancy.[5,7–9] Life expectancy among those with schizophrenia is 20% shorter compared with the general population,[4,5] and mental health consumers die 25 years younger than those with no mental illnesses.[9,10] This excessive mortality is currently viewed as a mortality crisis by mental health policy makers and researchers.[11(p49)]

Psychiatric nurses can provide leadership in using evidence-based research to improve the physical health of people with schizophrenia. The purpose of this article is to describe what is currently known about comorbid medical illnesses among adults and elderly people with schizophrenia; describe issues and trends in treatment and service delivery, and discuss the implications of current treatment for psychiatric nurses.

Multiple factors contribute to the development of medical problems in people with schizophrenia. The high prevalence of metabolic and cardiovascular abnormalities has been attributed to lifestyle factors and unhealthy behaviors that

---

[a] University of Kentucky College of Nursing, 202 College of Nursing Building, 760 Rose Street, Lexington, KY 40536-0232, USA
[b] Baptist Hospital East, Crisis Management Unit, 4000 Kresge Way, Louisville, KY 40207, USA
* Corresponding author.
E-mail address: peggy.el-mallakh@uky.edu

Nurs Clin N Am 45 (2010) 591–611
doi:10.1016/j.cnur.2010.06.008
0029-6465/10/$ – see front matter

increase the risk for development of chronic medical illnesses, such as smoking, poor diet, and lack of exercise.[12–16] Research findings indicate that up to 90% of people with schizophrenia smoke, compared with about 23% in the general population.[17,18] Dietary intake is often unhealthy as a result of food choices that are high in saturated fats and carbohydrates,[19] and rates of obesity are estimated to range from 40% to 62% among those with schizophrenia[12] People with schizophrenia often lack the skills to select and cook healthy foods, which results in poor nutrition and weight gain.[15] Because of a lack of adequate financial resources to purchase healthy foods, they may rely on food banks,[20] and these resources often have limited availability of healthy foods, such as whole grains and fresh fruit and vegetables. Furthermore, individuals with schizophrenia are often sedentary[13,21]; a study that used accelerometers to measure physical activity among 55 adults with severe mental illnesses found that only 4% achieved the level of physical activity recommended by the Surgeon General, and none of the participants who were overweight or obese met the recommended levels.[22]

Recent research indicates that the use of antipsychotic medications is associated with metabolic and cardiovascular abnormalities in people with schizophrenia. Traditional, first-generation, antipsychotic medications, such as chlorpromazine, perphenazine, and thioridazine often cause weight gain because of their antihistaminic potency.[23] Similarly, clinical research has yielded much information about the potential for weight gain with the use of atypical antipsychotics with antihistaminic potency, such as olanzapine, clozapine, and quetiapine. Additional research has been conducted to assess metabolic and cardiovascular abnormalities associated with the use of antipsychotic medications in the Clinical Antipsychotic Trials of Intervention Effectiveness (CATIE) study,[24–26] the Comparison of Atypicals for First Episode (CAFE) study,[27] and the European Cardiovascular, Lipid and Metabolic Outcomes Research in Schizophrenia (CLAMORS) study.[28–32]

Research suggests that gender may play a role in negative health outcomes among those with schizophrenia who are treated with atypical antipsychotic medications.[33] According to Seeman,[33] women have more fatty tissue per body weight compared with men; because atypical antipsychotic medications are lipophilic, negative health outcomes may be attributed to higher levels of drugs accumulating in fatty tissues of women diagnosed with schizophrenia. Consequently, women with schizophrenia treated with atypical antipsychotics have an increased risk for weight gain, development of diabetes, more severe dyslipidemia, higher rates of metabolic syndrome, higher rates of QT prolongation, and more frequent clozapine-induced agranulocytosis.

In general, elderly people with schizophrenia are an understudied population, and little research has been conducted to examine issues of comorbid medical illnesses in this population. One study compared general medical conditions among younger (age <60 years, n = 5859) and older (age ≥60 years, n = 2224) veterans with schizophrenia; findings suggest that older veterans were more likely to be diagnosed with cardiovascular conditions, particularly hypertension, congestive heart failure, peripheral vascular disease, and stroke.[34] In addition, older veterans were more likely to be diagnosed with endocrine diseases compared with younger veterans, particularly diabetes. The investigators attribute the higher incidence of these medical illnesses in people with schizophrenia to the chronic overactivity of physiologic process associated with a diagnosis of schizophrenia, which can be conceptualized as "'wear and tear' on the body and brain"[34(p253)] resulting from the need to adapt to environmental stressors triggered by the presence of a severe mental illness.

The presence of comorbid chronic conditions in the elderly schizophrenia popula-tion often go undiagnosed or do not receive appropriate care.[35] In addition, some comorbidities and unique characteristics of the elderly with schizophrenia are associ-ated with reduced functioning and motivation. Current research indicates that depres-sion is the most common comorbid condition among this population.[1,35,36] As the quantity of comorbid conditions increases with age, the severity of depressive symp-toms also increases.[1] In addition, older adults with schizophrenia have been shown to participate in fewer public and private leisure activities and leave their houses less often than the general population.[37] This population has also been shown to have lower income, smaller social networks, poorer daily functioning, and higher incidences of suicidal ideation than the comparison group.[36] There is evidence of illness improve-ment and stabilization with increasing age, although cognitive deficits seem to be exacerbated by age-related decline.[38] Elderly women with schizophrenia are also believed to have a greater decline in functioning than men as this population ages; the reason for this is not yet clear.[35] Depression, isolation, reduction in functioning, and exacerbated cognitive decline have the potential to interfere with patients' ability to care for complex chronic medical illnesses, such as diabetes. Although the current population of elderly persons with schizophrenia is small, it is projected to drastically increase in the future. As treatments for younger adults with schizophrenia improve, so their life expectancy improves,[39] and the potential for developing chronic medical illnesses. Further research must focus on older adults with schizophrenia, and the issues unique to this population.

OVERVIEW OF MEDICAL ILLNESSES IN PEOPLE WITH SCHIZOPHRENIA
Metabolic Syndrome

Metabolic syndrome is characterized by the co-occurrence of several metabolic abnormalities, including abdominal obesity and increased triglyceride levels, fasting serum glucose level, and hypertension.[39] Risk factors for developing metabolic syndrome include a high-fat diet, physical inactivity, family history of premature cardiovascular disease, and smoking.[40] The dyslipidemia and metabolic abnormalities that characterize metabolic syndrome are associated with high rates of atheroscle-rotic cardiovascular disease and type 2 diabetes mellitus (T2DM). Lifestyle interven-tions, such as aerobic exercise and weight loss, can reduce insulin resistance and dyslipidemia associated with metabolic syndrome. Pharmacologic treatment typically includes statins and antihypertensive agents.[39]

Mental health consumers frequently have several lifestyle risk factors associated with the development of metabolic syndrome, particularly obesity and physical inac-tivity. However, treatment of psychosis with atypical antipsychotic medications pres-ents an additional risk for metabolic syndrome. Among the 1460 CATIE study participants, almost 41% had the constellation of abnormalities associated with meta-bolic syndrome; 51.6% were men and 36% were women.[30] However, among the 1452 CLAMORS study participants, 24.6% had metabolic syndrome; of these, 23.6% were men and 27.2% were women.[28] Other studies have reported rates of 28.4% to 37.3%.[41,42]

The CATIE and CAFE studies have identified trends in the development of metabolic syndrome among participants treated with atypical antipsychotic medications. In the CATIE study, 34.8% of participants treated with olanzapine (n = 164) at baseline met the diagnostic criteria for metabolic syndrome, compared with almost 44% at 3 months. In comparison, rates of metabolic syndrome increased slightly in the group treated with perphenazine, and decreased in the ziprasidone and quetiapine groups.[31]

No changes in rates of metabolic syndrome were seen in the group treated with risperidone. The CAFE study suggests that metabolic syndrome develops in young patients treated with atypical antipsychotic medications after 1 year of treatment. The researchers investigated the metabolic effects of olanzapine, quetiapine, and risperidone among 400 participants with "early psychosis,"[27(p13)] defined as a diagnosis of schizophrenia, schizophreniform, or schizoaffective disorder for 1 month to 5 years. Findings indicate that 13.4% developed metabolic syndrome at the end of the first year of the study; of these participants, 22 were treated with olanzapine, 18 with quetiapine, and 11 with risperidone.[27]

Diabetes Mellitus

Diabetes mellitus (DM), a serious and chronic endocrine disorder, is "characterized by hyperglycemia resulting from defects in insulin secretion, insulin action, or both."[43(pS42)] Approximately 90% to 95% of diagnosed cases are type 2 DM, characterized by progressive defects in insulin secretion and insulin resistance resulting from obesity. The goals of treatment of T2DM are maintenance of glycosylated hemoglobin (HbA1C) levels of <7%,[43] and prevention of both short- and long-term complications of abnormal glucose levels.[44] Treatment consists of oral hypoglycemic agents, dietary modifications, weight management, and regular physical activity.[43] However, approximately 30% to 34% of patients diagnosed with T2DM require treatment with insulin in addition to oral hypoglycemic agents to maintain HbA1C levels of <7%.[45]

High prevalence rates of DM among mental health consumers with schizophrenia have been well documented.[6,46–48] Among those with schizophrenia, approximately 15% to 18% have a comorbid diagnosis of T2DM, and up to 30% have impaired glucose tolerance.[49] In contrast, the Centers for Disease Control[50] estimates that approximately 7% of the general population in the United States has a diagnosis of T2DM.

People diagnosed with schizophrenia face unique challenges in engaging in diabetes self-care activities because of sociodemographic characteristics, symptoms of psychosis, cognitive functioning, and additional comorbidities associated with schizophrenia.[51–53] A research study investigating medication adherence among 11,454 veterans with schizophrenia and T2DM found that substance abuse, comorbid depression, African American ethnicity, and homelessness were associated with lower adherence to medications for T2DM.[54] However, findings from this study also indicated that increased adherence was associated with more outpatient visits, lower copayments for medications, receiving medications in the mail, and more complex medication regimens. Additional research suggests that diabetes knowledge is low among those with schizophrenia and diabetes, particularly related to diet.[52] Furthermore, a study comparing cognitive functioning in people with schizophrenia and diabetes, diabetes only, and schizophrenia only found that cognitive impairments among those with schizophrenia and diabetes were significantly lower compared with the schizophrenia-only and diabetes-only groups. In addition, more cognitive deficits were associated with longer duration of diabetes, age of onset, and worse glycemic control. These cognitive deficits can potentially interfere with information processing and problem-solving ability required for adequate diabetes self-management.[51]

Cardiovascular

Research indicates that cardiovascular disease is 1 of the leading causes of death among those with serious mental illnesses[24,55]; up to 66% of people with schizophrenia die as a result of coronary heart disease, compared with 50% in the general population.[56,57] Several cardiovascular abnormalities are associated with metabolic syndrome, particularly increased triglyceride levels and hypertension.[28,58,59] Sachs[58] reports that a diagnosis of metabolic syndrome is associated with a 4-fold increase in mortality from coronary heart disease.

Cardiovascular disease in people with schizophrenia may be linked to the use of atypical antipsychotic medication because of medication-induced insulin resistance and consequent increased triglyceride and low-density lipoprotein (LDL) cholesterol levels.[29,31,59,60] For example, the CATIE study found that among 246 participants, nonfasting triglycerides were increased between baseline and 3 months, and the greatest increases were seen for participants treated with quetiapine and olanzapine.[31] Similarly, the CATIE researchers examined the development of 10-year cardiovascular disease risk among 1125 of the study participants.[29] Markers indicating an increased 10-year risk for developing coronary heart disease were seen in participants treated with quetiapine and olanzapine; participants treated with perphenazine, risperidone, and ziprasidone showed a decreased 10-year risk for the development of coronary heart disease.

Obesity

Obesity, defined as body mass index ≥ 30 kg/m^2,[61] greatly increases the risk for metabolic and cardiovascular abnormalities common among those with schizophrenia, particularly metabolic syndrome, hypertension, T2DM, and coronary heart disease. Risk factors for obesity include a high-fat, high-sugar diet, and physical inactivity. Obesity is a highly prevalent metabolic abnormality among people with schizophrenia, particularly among women. Studies have shown that approximately 30% of men with schizophrenia are obese, compared with about 60% of women with schizophrenia.[7,62–64] The relationship between a diagnosis of schizophrenia and obesity is unclear. Although research suggests that obesity is a common side effect of atypical antipsychotic medication use, particularly olanzapine,[5] others have observed that obesity occurs in some newly diagnosed patients who have never been treated with atypical antipsychotic medications.[7]

Research related to diet in this population has yielded varying results. Henderson and colleagues[12] compared dietary intake profiles among 88 patients with schizophrenia to a control group from the National Health and Nutrition Examination Survey; participants were matched on age, gender, and ethnicity. Findings indicate that the mean body mass index (BMI, calculated as weight in kilograms divided by the square of height in meters) of study participants was significantly higher than the matched controls. However, those with schizophrenia consumed significantly fewer overall calories, carbohydrates, protein, fats, and micronutrients, and significantly more caffeine, than the matched controls. The investigators suggest that the findings could be attributed to the use of antipsychotic medications and lack of physical activity in the sample participants diagnosed with schizophrenia.

Pulmonary

Smoking is a significant concern among people with schizophrenia. People with schizophrenia smoke for many reasons, including boredom, coping with stress and anxiety, controlling negative symptoms and side effects of medications, and because their friends smoke.[17,65] According to Grant and Keltner,[66] nicotine increases synaptic dopamine, and people with schizophrenia may smoke to compensate for down-regulation of dopamine expression and receptor binding in the limbic and prefrontal cortical areas of the brain. Thus, smoking stimulates dopamine activity in the areas of the brain that improve mood, sharpen cognition, and decrease appetite.[66] Yet the consequences of smoking in this population are both severe and avoidable.

This modifiable behavior increases the likelihood of cardiac-related mortality in this population[55,67] Kelly and colleagues[67] investigated the risk of smoking-related adverse outcomes among 1213 people, aged 19 to 69 years, who were diagnosed with schizophrenia. Findings indicated that among those aged 35 to 54 years, cardiac-related mortality was 12 times higher compared with nonsmokers. Some interventions to help patients reduce smoking or achieve abstinence seem promising. Evins and colleagues[18] conducted a 12-week study to compare bupropion with placebo in combination with nicotine replacement therapy and cognitive behavioral therapy for smoking cessation among 51 smokers with schizophrenia. Findings suggest that the group that received bupropion had higher smoking reduction and abstinence rates compared with placebo.

CURRENT INITIATIVES IN INTERVENTION RESEARCH

Current intervention research is focused on optimizing a variety of health outcomes among those with serious mental illnesses, including schizophrenia spectrum disorders (SSDs).[13,68–75] Several research studies have been conducted to determine the effectiveness of health and wellness promotion interventions; these include weight loss programs, smoking cessation, wellness and healthy living, physical activity programs, and diabetes self-management skills training. A summary of recent research is presented in **Table 1**.

ACCESS TO CARE ISSUES

High prevalence rates of medical illnesses among people with schizophrenia have been extensively researched and reported, and current initiatives are in progress to expand the evidence base to improve the treatment of those with comorbid illnesses. However, despite the knowledge base and practice guideline development efforts, health service use research indicates that access to medical treatment for these illnesses is inadequate. Rates of monitoring for medical problems and hospitalizations are low among people with schizophrenia.[32,76–78] Haupt and colleagues[76] note that in 2004, the American Diabetes Association (ADA) issued guidelines for metabolic monitoring for people treated with atypical antipsychotic medications. They compared rates of metabolic and cardiovascular monitoring among patients enrolled in 70 managed-care programs, both before and after the guidelines were established. Findings indicate that although rates of monitoring for metabolic and cardiovascular problems increased significantly after the ADA guidelines were established, overall rates of monitoring remained low. Before the guidelines were issued, rates of lipid monitoring among 5787 people were 8.4% at baseline and 6.8% at 12 weeks; rates of glucose monitoring were 17.3% at baseline and 14.1% at 12 weeks. Following the establishment of the ADA guidelines, rates of lipid monitoring among 17,832 people with schizophrenia were 10.5% at baseline and 9.0% at 12 weeks; rates of glucose testing were 21.8% at baseline and 17.9% at 12 weeks.

Similarly, Nasrallah and colleagues[32] found low rates of treatment of metabolic and cardiovascular problems among 1460 participants in the CATIE study. They report that 30.2% of participants with diabetes, 62.4% with hypertension, and 88% with dyslipidemia were not receiving treatment for their medical problems at the time they enrolled in the CATIE study. In a study by Himelhoch and colleagues,[77] smokers and nonsmokers with schizophrenia and T2DM were significantly less likely to be treated with statins and angiotensin-converting enzyme inhibitors. They also received less frequent lipid monitoring compared with smokers and nonsmokers with T2DM and no diagnosis of schizophrenia. Kilbourne and colleagues[78] found that in the

Veteran's Administration health care system, patients with serious mental illnesses and diabetes were less likely to receive retinal examinations, renal testing, and foot examinations compared with patients with no comorbid psychiatric diagnosis.

Disparities in treatment among those with schizophrenia have prompted clinicians and policy makers to express serious concerns about the links between inadequate treatment, excessive mortality, and reduced life expectancy among people with schizophrenia.[8,11] Gittelman[8] maintains that life expectancy is short in this population as a result of inadequate care for physical illnesses. Manderscheid and Delvecchio[10] concur, stating that mental health consumers "are dying from untreated high blood pressure and stroke, untreated diabetes, untreated chronic heart disease, the direct consequences of smoking ... and the unintended consequences of the metabolic side effects designed to address psychiatric illnesses".[(p.3)] In addition to increased morbidity and mortality, medical illnesses are associated with poor quality of life[6] and interfere with recovery efforts in those with mental health problems.[79]

The National Association of State Mental Health Program Directors (NASMHPD)[79] has called for improved access to high-quality health care and comprehensive initiatives in the public mental health system to reduce morbidity and mortality among mental health consumers with schizophrenia and comorbid medical illnesses. NASMHPD's goal is to implement strategies recommended by the Institute of Medicine[80] for the purpose of providing safe, effective, patient-centered, timely, efficient, and equitable health care to mental health consumers in the public mental health services system. One proposed strategy is the establishment of standard health indicators that are systematically monitored in state mental health service systems. In addition, NASMHPD recommends the dissemination and implementation of the Chronic Care Model (CCM)[81] in publicly funded mental health systems to deliver "continuous, planned care"[(p.6)] to mental health consumers with comorbid medical illnesses. The CCM includes decision support for clinicians, patient-centered illness management education, comprehensive care management, measurement of performance indicators, and monitoring of evidence-based care protocols.[79] Furthermore, NASMHPD contends that other essential strategies include enhanced collaboration between providers, peer-directed prevention activities, improved access to dental care, and expanded Medicaid financing for primary prevention and health promotion services such as weight loss and smoking cessation programs. Everett and colleagues[82] stress that the structure of financing for medical services in a psychiatric setting must be adapted to eliminate barriers to reimbursement, and further state that "Medicare and Medicaid must become partners in improving access to care, data analysis, and designing and implementing strategies that will be effective with the population served by the public mental health system".[(p.21)]

IMPLICATIONS FOR NURSES

The current state of medical problems among people with schizophrenia has several implications for nursing practice and research.

Practice

Psychiatric nurses are challenged to provide care that optimizes health outcomes in people with schizophrenia and comorbid medical illnesses. In clinical practice settings, particularly inpatient units, maintaining competency in assessing and intervening for complications of metabolic and cardiovascular abnormalities is essential. In addition, psychiatric nurses can intervene to reduce risk for development of

Table 1
Summary of intervention studies to improve health outcomes in people with schizophrenia

Reference	Sample	Treatment Groups	Intervention	Intensity and Duration	Outcomes	Findings
Beebe et al,[13] 2005	Diagnosis: 100% SSDs Age range: 40–63 y % male: 80% Setting: outpatient	T = 4 C = 6	Walk-Address-Learn-Cue (WALC): walking program, education about exercise, stretching exercises	Treadmill exercise 3 times per week for 16 wk	BMI Levels of aerobic fitness % body fat Psychiatric symptoms	Treatment group had significant reduction in body fat Treatment group had nonsignificant reduction in BMI, positive and negative symptoms, and higher level of aerobic fitness compared with control group
Menza et al,[68] 2004	Diagnosis: 100% SSDs C = 100% SSDs Mean age: T = 42.6 C = 47.2 % male T = 61% C = 50% Setting: Day treatment programs	T = 31 C = 20	Healthy Living: multimodal approach; nutrition, exercise, behavioral interventions	12 wk of twice weekly intensive groups/ weekly individual sessions; 12 wk of less intensive weekly groups/weekly individual sessions; 6 mo of weekly weight maintenance groups/ monthly individual session; total 52 wk	Primary: BMI; weight Secondary: HbA1C, systolic and diastolic blood pressure, exercise per week; nutrition knowledge; cholesterol; triglycerides	Treatment group: significant decrease in BMI and weight; significant improvements in HbA1C, systolic and diastolic BP; exercise, nutrition knowledge; no significant changes in cholesterol or triglycerides Control group gained weight

Study	Sample	Intervention	Duration	Outcomes Measured	Results
Kwon et al,[69] 2006	Diagnosis: 100% SSDs Mean age: T = 32 ± 9.22 y C = 29.8 ± 6.07 y % male: T = 30% C = 33.3% Setting: 4 clinical centers	Diet and exercise management; lifestyle modifications	Weekly for 4 wk, biweekly for 8 wk, total 12 wk	Weight; BMI; quality of life; safety (vital signs)	Significant weight loss seen at week 8 and reduction in BMI at week 12 for treatment and control groups Nonsignificant reduction in LDL/HDL ratio in treatment group; nonsignificant reductions in systolic BP, diastolic BP and pulse between treatment and control groups
T = 33 C = 15					
McKibbin et al,[70] 2006	Diagnosis: T = 100% SSDs C = 100% SSDs Mean age: T = 53.1 ± 10.4 C = 54.8 ± 8.2 % male: T = 68% C = 62% Setting: outpatient	Diabetes Awareness and Rehabilitation Training: glucometer use; DM complications, diet, exercise, foot care	Weekly 90-min sessions for 24 wk	Weight; BMI; systolic and diastolic blood pressure; fasting blood glucose; HbA1C; cholesterol; diabetes knowledge; diabetes self-efficacy; physical activity	Treatment group had significant reductions in weight, BMI, triglycerides compared with control group No significant differences in fasting blood glucose, HbA1C, cholesterol Treatment group had significant improvements in diabetes knowledge and slight increase in diabetes self-efficacy; control group had decreased diabetes self-efficacy
T = 28 C = 29					

(continued on next page)

Table 1 (continued)						
Reference	Sample	Treatment Groups	Intervention	Intensity and Duration	Outcomes	Findings
Chiverton et al,[71] 2007	Diagnosis: 46% SSDs Mean age: 46 y % male: 32.4% Setting: outpatient	T = 74 No control group	Well-Balanced Program: medications, glucometer, nutrition, physical activity, stress management, skin, foot, eye care; screening and community resources	Weekly nursing intervention visits for 16 wk	Health risk status HbA1C Client satisfaction	Significant improvement in health risk status Significant decrease in HbA1C High satisfaction scores
Chafetz et al,[72] 2008	Diagnosis: T = 35% SSDs C = 31% SSDs Mean age: T = 38 y (10.2) C = 38.5 y (10.0) % male T = 68.4% C = 67.5% Setting: short-term residential treatment	T = 155 C = 154	Wellness training added to basic primary care: current health status; rating importance of health status; psychiatric symptoms that affect health; physical symptoms and health problems; personal strategies to manage problems; planning for health	Flexible schedule for use of wellness resources for up to 12 mo	Perceived health status Health-related self-efficacy Psychosocial functioning	Treatment group: intervention was significantly associated with improvement in physical functioning, self-reported general health status, controlling for severity of illness and drug/alcohol use No significant changes in health-related self-efficacy or psychosocial functioning

| Lindenmayer et al,[73] 2009 | Diagnosis: 79% SSDs Mean age: 44.25 y (10.87) Setting: inpatient; rehabilitative treatment mall | T = 402 No control group | Solutions for Wellness and Team Solutions: medication education, symptoms of mental illness, recovery promotion, relapse prevention, nutrition, fitness, practice exercise | 3-level structured education program of 50 min, twice daily; level 1: 4 wk of assessment, 12 wk program; level 2: 16 wk of program; level 3: 16 wk of program | Knowledge assessments; weight, BMI, triglycerides, cholesterol; HbA1C | Significant weight loss over time; significant reduction in BMI for participants whose baseline BMI was ≥30 kg/m^2; significant reductions in glucose and triglyceride levels No significant changes in HbA1C, HDL cholesterol, LDL cholesterol Significant correlations seen between weight and Fitness/Exercise knowledge score; significant correlations seen between glucose levels and Nutrition/ Healthy Lifestyle knowledge score |

(continued on next page)

Table 1
(continued)

Reference	Sample	Treatment Groups	Intervention	Intensity and Duration	Outcomes	Findings
Van Citters et al,[74] 2009	Diagnosis: 24% SSDs Mean age: 43.5 ± 11.4 y % men: 28% Setting: outpatient; community integrated	T = 76 No control group	In SHAPE Program: individualized health promotion and education, focused on healthy eating and exercise; health mentor and participant collaborate to develop individualized health promotion plan; weekly meetings with health mentor; free access to local fitness organizations; group-based fitness and nutrition sessions	Weekly meeting with health mentor for 9 mo	Physical activity; readiness to change weight loss/dietary behaviors; weight, BMI, systolic/ diastolic BP; physical/mental health functioning	Significant increases in hours spent exercising, vigorous and leisure physical activity, reduced waist circumference, improved mental health functioning No significant changes in BMI, systolic/ diastolic BP or physical functioning Low engagement in dietary behavior changes

| Druss et al,[75] 2010 | Diagnosis:
T: 26.8% SSDs
C = 31% SSDs
Mean age:
T = 47.8 ± 10.1 y
C = 48.4 ± 10.1 y
X% male
T = 34%
C = 25.6%
Setting: outpatient | T = 41
C = 39 | Health and Recovery Peer Program (HARP): groups led by peer specialists; self-management overview, exercise/physical activity; pain/fatigue management; healthy eating on a limited budget; medication management; finding and working with a regular doctor | Up to 6 group sessions led by mental health peer specialists | Patient activation (perceived ability to manage illness/health behaviors and act as an effective patient)
Disease self-management (physical activity, health service use, medication adherence)
Health-related quality of life | Treatment group had significantly higher levels of activation and health-related quality of life (physical component) at 6 mo compared with control group
Treatment group had nonsignificant higher levels of exercise compared with control group
Treatment group had 14.2% increase in medication adherence
Control group had 7.3% decline in medication adherence |

Abbreviations: BP, blood pressure; C, control; HDL, high-density lipoprotein; LDL, low-density lipoprotein; SSDs, schizophrenia spectrum disorders; T, treatment.

comorbid medical problems by providing health promotion education to their clients. Wellness and exercise groups can be implemented both on inpatient units and community mental health settings to teach healthy living practices and encourage physical activity. Smoking cessation counseling and support groups are essential to reduce the high mortality associated with this risky behavior.[83] Keltner and Grant[66] stress that mental health clinicians need to be vigilant in assessing patients undergoing smoking cessation therapy, because psychiatric symptoms may be exacerbated or covered up by symptoms of nicotine withdrawal.

Psychiatric nurses play a critical role in assisting patients with illness management. People with schizophrenia often face unique problems in managing their illnesses, particularly diabetes; for example, patients often do not know how to cook and do not have money to purchase healthy foods. They may rely heavily on inexpensive fast food and pre-prepared microwavable foods, which frequently have a high salt and fat content. Nutrition education is needed to teach patients how to read food labels, determine portion sizes, and select healthy food choices that are within their budget. Furthermore, patients need to know about community resources such as food banks. Nurses should also assess patients' ability to complete other diabetes self-care activities, such as glucometer testing and medication administration. Because of cognitive impairments, patients may have difficulty interpreting the results of glucometer testing and adjusting insulin doses based on the results. In addition, severe hand tremors caused by side effects of some psychotropic medications can interfere with diabetes self-care activities; tremors make it difficult for them to use a lancet to obtain a blood sample, draw up the blood droplet into a test strip, insert the strip into a glucometer, and self-administer an insulin injection. Nurses should assess patients' ability to engage in these illness management activities and if needed, recommend family support or Visiting Nurses Association to provide assistance to patients with their self-care activities. Education on diabetes self-management and healthy living can also be provided by inpatient or community-based nurses; the National Diabetes Education Program has several easy-to-read self-care manuals and educational materials that nurses can use in individual or group counseling sessions.

Adequate treatment of medical comorbidities is critically important to promote the overall health and functioning of those with schizophrenia, and advanced practice psychiatric nurses play an integral role in the treatment of people with comorbidities. Research has identified several practice guidelines and recommendations for screening and monitoring medical comorbidities and prescribing medications.[24,40,56,83–85] For patients who want to quit smoking, bupropion SR, with or without nicotine replacement therapy, is recommended to achieve short-term smoking abstinence.[83] However, caution must be used when prescribing bupropion, which is metabolized by CYP 2D6, when the patient is being treated with CYP 2D6 inhibitors or inducers.[86] For patients with medical and cardiac comorbidities, initial assessment and annual follow-ups should include a complete medical history, weight, BMI, electrocardiogram, comprehensive laboratory tests, other relevant tests, and assessment of patient knowledge about health behaviors.[24] When initiating treatment with either a traditional first-generation or an atypical second-generation antipsychotic medication, baseline and ongoing monitoring should include weight, waist circumference, BMI, blood pressure, lipids (total cholesterol, LDL cholesterol, high-density lipoprotein [HDL] cholesterol, triglycerides), fasting serum glucose, and/or HbA1C.[87] Close follow-up monitoring of weight in the first months of treatment is critical; according to McElroy,[62] rapid weight gain in the first month of treatment may be a risk factor for further substantial weight gain.(p.15)

Atypical antipsychotic medications are an effective treatment strategy for schizophrenia, despite the undesirable metabolic and cardiovascular side effects.[83,88] Brunero and colleagues[89] maintain that the risk of metabolic problems should be balanced by the effectiveness of atypical antipsychotics, such as clozapine, in treating positive and negative symptoms of schizophrenia. Practice guidelines have been developed for the strategic use of atypical antipsychotic medications in mental health consumers who are at risk for developing comorbid medical problems. For example, some clinicians recommend selection of medications that minimize the risk for weight gain and abnormal metabolic and cardiovascular side effects.[40,90] Weiden[91] maintains that for patients treated with medications that have significant metabolic and cardiovascular side effects, switching to an alternative medication with comparable efficacy but lower risk for side effects can promote weight loss and reduce the risk of dyslipidemia in some patients. However, patient preference, previous response, and side effects of previous medications should be considered when selecting an antipsychotic medication.[40]

In general, clinicians and researchers recommend integrated treatment models for providing care to people with schizophrenia and complex health care needs; this involves a multidisciplinary team approach with collaboration between psychiatric and primary care providers.[24,84,92] Clinicians stress the need for establishing a designated provider who is responsible for the patient's medical care, including oversight of monitoring metabolic and cardiovascular status. If providers of psychiatric treatment do not provide medical care to their patients, they must be vigilant for the presence of medical comorbidities, monitor for metabolic and cardiovascular side effects at each service encounter, and refer to medical providers when indicated.[85,93] In addition, effective communication between primary care clinicians and members of the treatment team is crucial.[85,92]

At the advanced practice level, collaboration between family nurse practitioners and advanced practice psychiatric nurses is crucial to effectively coordinate the treatment of complex medical problems in this population. Advanced practice nursing education can further facilitate practitioners' ability to promote optimal health outcomes by incorporating principles of multidisciplinary teamwork and collaboration into advanced practice curricula. In addition, faculty in advanced practice education programs can emphasize the use of established models for chronic illness care, such as the CCM, in integrated treatment settings.

Research

Findings from preliminary research to improve the wellness and health outcomes of those with comorbid illnesses and schizophrenia are encouraging. Researchers stress the need for continued longitudinal research to investigate the effectiveness of health promotion and illness management interventions for this population. In addition, ongoing research is needed to clarify the unique issues that can influence treatment adherence and health outcomes in people with schizophrenia, such as cognitive impairments and functioning. Based on the research related to those diagnosed with only physical illnesses and no comorbid psychiatric illnesses, these factors likely include family support, health literacy, motivation to engage in health behaviors, health beliefs, self-efficacy, psychosocial adjustment to chronic illnesses, and illness-related distress.[93] Research to identify the relationships among these factors in people with schizophrenia is critically important to improve health outcomes.

Currently, mental health research focuses primarily on the relationships between pharmacologic treatment and metabolic and cardiovascular outcomes, prevention efforts, and treatment models that optimize access to appropriate evidence-based care. However, emerging theories in social epidemiology suggest that the broader societal context, such as socioeconomic status, contributes significantly to health disparities in vulnerable populations. For example, chronic conditions such as diabetes and cardiovascular disease are more prevalent among people with low educational attainment, low literacy, unemployment, and low socioeconomic position. Among people with diabetes, low socioeconomic status is associated with increased risk of morbidity and mortality.[94–96]

People with schizophrenia frequently experience stigma, marginalization, and discrimination in housing and employment as a result of cognitive impairments, treatment refractory symptoms, and poor functioning,[80] and they frequently live in poverty or are homeless.[97,98] It is likely that chronic stress associated with unemployment, poverty, marginalization, isolation, and stigma is linked to poor physical health in this population. In addition, poverty prevents people with schizophrenia and comorbid medical problems from obtaining food, medications, and other resources necessary to successfully engage in self-care for their medical illnesses.[20] Additional research is needed to examine the relationships between social determinants of health, constraints to self-care, and the physical health status of people with schizophrenia.

SUMMARY

The physical health of people with schizophrenia is poor, and the challenges in finding effective treatment and optimizing health outcomes are significant. However, it is likely that people diagnosed with schizophrenia can be partners in the treatment of their physical health problems. Research suggests that many people with schizophrenia value physical health and will participate in health-related behaviors when they are provided with the opportunity to do so.[99]

A review of the literature reveals a distinct pattern in the epidemiology and treatment of physical illnesses: high prevalence rates of chronic and potentially fatal illnesses, and low rates of treatment of these illnesses. The need for improvement in the availability of medical care for people with schizophrenia is urgent[85,90,100]; practice guidelines based on the most rigorous research evidence are useless if people with schizophrenia cannot access services. Maj[100] asserts that "[i]f we want to state convincingly that we care about our patients' quality of life and civil rights, we must make promotion of physical health care a priority".[(p.13)] Both psychiatric and primary care health care providers must be active in advocacy, education, and research to address disparities in medical treatment for people with schizophrenia, and enhance the evidence base to optimize treatment and health outcomes.

REFERENCES

1. Chwastiak LA, Rosenheck RA, McEvoy JP, et al. Interrelationships of psychiatric symptom severity, medical comorbidity, and functioning in schizophrenia. Psychiatr Serv 2006;57(8):1102–9.
2. Cimpean D, Torrey WC, Green AI. Schizophrenia and co-occurring general medical illness. Psychiatr Ann 2005;35(1):71–81.
3. Batki SL, Meszaros ZS, Strutynski K, et al. Medical comorbidity in patients with schizophrenia and alcohol dependence. Schizophr Res 2009;107:139–46.
4. Fagiolini A, Goracci A. The effects of undertreated chronic medical illnesses in patients with severe mental disorders. J Clin Psychiatry 2009;70(Suppl 3):22–9.
5. Hennekens CH. Increasing global burden of cardiovascular disease in general populations and patients with schizophrenia. J Clin Psychiatry 2007;68 (Suppl 4):4–7.

6. Howard PB, El-Mallakh P, Rayens MK, et al. Comorbid medical illnesses and perceived general health among adult recipients of Medicaid mental health services. Issues Ment Health Nurs 2007;28:255–74.
7. Allison DB, Newcomer JW, Dunn AL, et al. Obesity among those with mental disorders: a National Institute of Mental Health meeting report. Am J Prev Med 2009;36(4):341–50.
8. Gittelman M. Why are the mentally ill dying? Int J Ment Health 2008;37(1):3–12.
9. Manderscheid RW. Premature death among state mental health agency consumers: assessing progress in addressing a quiet tragedy. Int J Public Health 2009;54:1–2.
10. Manderscheid RW, Delvecchio P. Moving toward solutions: responses to the crisis of premature death. Int J Ment Health 2008;37(2):3–7.
11. Manderscheid RW, Druss B, Freeman E. Data to manage the mortality crisis. Int J Ment Health 2008;37(2):49–68.
12. Henderson DC, Borba CP, Daley TB, et al. Dietary intake profile of patients with schizophrenia. Ann Clin Psychiatry 2006;18(2):99–105.
13. Beebe LH, Tian L, Morris N, et al. Effects of exercise on mental and physical health parameters of persons with schizophrenia. Issues Ment Health Nurs 2005;26:661–76.
14. Dixon L, Weiden P, Delahanty J, et al. Prevalence and correlates of diabetes in national schizophrenia samples. Schizophr Bull 2000;26(4):903–12.
15. Leas L, McCabe M. Health behaviors among individuals with schizophrenia and depression. J Health Psychol 2007;12(4):563–79.
16. Peet M. Diet, diabetes and schizophrenia: review and hypothesis. Br J Psychiatry 2004;184(Suppl 47):S102–5.
17. Esterberg ML, Compton MT. Smoking behavior in persons with a schizophrenia-spectrum disorder: a qualitative investigation of the transtheoretical model. Soc Sci Med 2005;61:293–303.
18. Evins AE, Cather C, Culhane MA, et al. A 12-week double-blind, placebo-controlled study of bupropion SR added to high-dose dual nicotine replacement therapy for smoking cessation or reduction in schizophrenia. J Clin Psychopharmacol 2007;27(4):380–6.
19. Henderson DC, Sharma B, Fan X, et al. Dietary saturated fat intake and glucose metabolism impairments in nondiabetic, nonobese patients with schizophrenia on clozapine or risperidone. Ann Clin Psychiatry 2010;22(1):33–42.
20. El-Mallakh P. Doing my best: poverty and self-care among individuals with schizophrenia and diabetes mellitus. Arch Psychiatr Nurs 2007;21(1):49–60.
21. Vreeland B. Bridging the gap between mental and physical health: a multidisciplinary approach. J Clin Psychiatry 2007;68(Suppl 4):26–33.
22. Jerome GJ, Young DR, Dalcin A, et al. Physical activity levels of persons with mental illness attending psychiatric rehabilitation programs. Schizophr Res 2009;108:252–7.
23. Barnett M, VonMuenster S, Wehring H, et al. Assessment of monitoring for glucose and lipid dysregulation in adult Medi-Cal patients newly started on antipsychotics. Ann Clin Psychiatry 2010;22(1):9–18.
24. Goff DG, Cather C, Evins AE, et al. Medical morbidity and mortality in schizophrenia: guidelines for psychiatrists. J Clin Psychiatry 2005;66:183–94.
25. Meyer JM, Davis VG, McEvoy JP, et al. Impact of antipsychotic treatment on nonfasting triglycerides in the CATIE schizophrenia trial phase 1. Schizophr Res 2008;103:104–9.

26. Stroup TS, McEvoy JP, Swartz MS, et al. The National Institute of Mental Health Clinical Antipsychotic Trials of Intervention Effectiveness [CATIE] project: schizophrenia trial design and protocol development. Schizophr Bull 2003; 29(1):15–31.

27. Patel JK, Buckley PF, Woolson S, et al. Metabolic profiles of second-generation antipsychotics in early psychosis: findings from the CAFE study. Schizophr Res 2009;111:9–16.

28. Bobes J, Arango C, Aranda P, et al. Cardiovascular and metabolic risk in outpatients with schizophrenia treated with antipsychotics: results of the CLAMORS study. Schizophr Res 2007;90:162–73.

29. Daumit GL, Goff DG, Meyer JM, et al. Antipsychotic effects on estimated 10-year coronary heart disease risk in the CATIE schizophrenia study. Schizophr Res 2008;105:175–87.

30. McEvoy JP, Meyer JM, Goff DC, et al. Prevalence of the metabolic syndrome in patients with schizophrenia: baseline results from the Clinical Antipsychotic Trials of Intervention Effectiveness (CATIE) schizophrenia trial and comparison with national estimates from NHANES III. Schizophr Res 2005;80:19–32.

31. Meyer JM, Davis VG, Goff DC, et al. Change in metabolic syndrome parameters with antipsychotic treatment in the CATIE schizophrenia trial: prospective data from phase 1. Schizophr Res 2008;101:273–86.

32. Nasrallah HA, Meyer JM, Goff DC, et al. Low rates of treatment for hypertension, dyslipidemia and diabetes in schizophrenia: data from the CATIE schizophrenia trial sample at baseline. Schizophr Res 2006;86:15–22.

33. Seeman MV. Schizophrenia: women bear a disproportionate toll of antipsychotic side effects. J Am Psychiatr Nurses Assoc 2010;16(1):21–9.

34. Kilbourne AM, Cornelius JR, Han X, et al. General-medical conditions in older patients with serious mental illness. Am J Geriatr Psychiatry 2005;13(3):250–4.

35. Karim S, Overshott R, Burns A. Older people with chronic schizophrenia. Aging Ment Health 2005;9(4):315–24.

36. Berry K, Barrowclough C. The needs of older adults with schizophrenia implications for psychological interventions. Clin Psychol Rev 2009;29:68–76.

37. Graham C, Arthur A, Howard R. The social functioning of older adults with schizophrenia. Aging Ment Health 2002;6(2):149–52.

38. Harvey PD. Cognitive and functional impairments in elderly patients with schizophrenia: a review of the recent literature. Harv Rev Psychiatry 2001; 9(2):59–68.

39. Cornier MA, Dabelea D, Hernandez TL, et al. The metabolic syndrome. Endocr Rev 2008;29(7):777–822.

40. Hasnain M, Viewveg WVR, Fredrickson SK, et al. Clinical monitoring and management of the metabolic syndrome in patients receiving atypical antipsychotic medications. Prim Care Diabetes 2009;3:5–15.

41. Correll CU, Frederickson AM, Kane JM, et al. Metabolic syndrome and the risk of coronary heart disease in 367 patients treated with second-generation antipsychotic drugs. J Clin Psychiatry 2006;67:575–83.

42. DeHert MA, van Winkel R, Van Eyck D, et al. Prevalence of the metabolic syndrome in patients with schizophrenia treated with antipsychotic medication. Schizophr Res 2006;83(1):87–93.

43. American Diabetes Association. Standards of medical care in diabetes—2007. Diabetes Care 2007;30(Suppl 1):S4–41.

44. Bethel MA, Feinglos MN. Basal insulin therapy in type 2 diabetes. J Am Board Fam Pract 2005;18:199–204.

45. Nelson SE, Palumbo PJ. Addition of insulin to oral therapy in patients with type 2 diabetes. Am J Med Sci 2006;331(5):257–63.
46. Bushe C, Holt R. Prevalence of diabetes and impaired glucose tolerance in patients with schizophrenia. Br J Psychiatry 2004;184(Suppl 47):S67–71.
47. Newcomer JW. Abnormalities of glucose metabolism associated with atypical antipsychotic drugs. J Clin Psychiatry 2004;65(Suppl 18):36–46.
48. Suvisaari J, Perala J, Saarni SI, et al. Type 2 diabetes among persons with schizophrenia and other psychotic disorders in a general population survey. Eur Arch Psychiatry Clin Neurosci 2007. Available at: www.springerlink.com. Accessed May 29, 2009.
49. Expert Group. 'Schizophrenia and diabetes 2003' expert consensus meeting, Dublin, 3-4 October 2003: consensus summary. Br J Psychiatry 2004;47:S112–4.
50. Center for Disease Control. National diabetes fact sheet, United States, 2005. Available at: http://www.cdc.gov/nchs/nhis.htm. Accessed October 17, 2009.
51. Dickerson D, Gold JM, Dickerson FB, et al. Evidence of exacerbated cognitive deficits in schizophrenia with comorbid diabetes. Psychosomatics 2008;49: 123–31.
52. Dickerson FB, Goldberg RW, Brown CH, et al. Diabetes knowledge among persons with serious mental illness and type 2 diabetes. Psychosomatics 2005;46:418–24.
53. El-Mallakh P. Evolving self-care in individuals with schizophrenia and diabetes mellitus. Arch Psychiatr Nurs 2006;20(2):55–64.
54. Kreyenbuhl J, Dixon LB, McCarthy JF, et al. Does adherence to medications for type 2 diabetes differ between individuals with vs. without schizophrenia? Schizophr Bull 2010;36(2):428–35.
55. Kilbourne AM, Morden NE, Austin K, et al. Excess heart-disease-related mortality in a national study of patients with mental disorders: identifying modifiable risk factors. Gen Hosp Psychiatry 2009;31:555–63.
56. Meyer JM. Strategies for the long-term treatment of schizophrenia: real-world lessons from the CATIE trial. J Clin Psychiatry 2007;68(Suppl 1):28–33.
57. Newcomer JW. Antipsychotic medications: metabolic and cardiovascular risk. J Clin Psychiatry 2007;68(Suppl 4):8–13.
58. Sachs FM. Metabolic syndrome: epidemiology and consequences. J Clin Psychiatry 2004;65(Suppl 18):3–12.
59. Stahl SM, Mignon L, Meyer JM. Which comes first: atypical antipsychotic treatment or cardiometabolic risk? Acta Psychiatr Scand 2009;119:171–9.
60. Casey DE. Dyslipidemia and atypical antipsychotic drugs. J Clin Psychiatry 2004;65(Suppl 18):27–35.
61. Ganguli R. Behavioral therapy for weight loss in patients with schizophrenia. J Clin Psychiatry 2007;68(Suppl 4):19–25.
62. McElroy SL. Obesity in patients with severe mental illness: overview and management. J Clin Psychiatry 2009;70(Suppl 3):12–21.
63. Wirshing D. Schizophrenia and obesity: impact of antipsychotic medications. J Clin Psychiatry 2004;65(Suppl 18):13–26.
64. McQuade RD, Stock E, Marcus R, et al. A comparison of weight change during treatment with olanzapine or aripiprazole: results from a randomized double-blind study. J Clin Psychiatry 2004;65(Suppl 18):47–56.
65. Forchuk C, Norman R, Malla A, et al. Schizophrenia and the motivation for smoking. Perspect Psychiatr Care 2002;38(2):41–9.
66. Keltner N, Grant JS. Smoke, smoke, smoke that cigarette. Perspect Psychiatr Care 2006;42(4):256–61.

67. Kelly DL, McMahon RP, Wehring HJ, et al. Cigarette smoking and mortality risk in people with schizophrenia. Schizophr Bull Dec 2009. [Epub ahead of print].

68. Menza M, Vreeland B, Minsky S, et al. Managing atypical antipsychotic-associated weight gain: 12-month data on a multimodal weight control program. J Clin Psychiatry 2004;65(4):471–7.

69. Kwon JS, Choi JS, Bakh WM, et al. Weight management program for treatment-emergent weight gain in olanzapine-treated patients with schizophrenia or schizoaffective disorder: a 12-week randomized controlled clinical trial. J Clin Psychiatry 2006;67:547–53.

70. McKibbin CL, Patterson TL, Norman G, et al. A lifestyle intervention for older schizophrenia patients with diabetes mellitus: a randomized controlled trial. Schizophr Res 2006;86:36–44.

71. Chiverton P, Lindley P, Tortoretti DM, et al. Well balanced: 8 steps to wellness for adults with mental illness and diabetes. J Psychosoc Nurs Ment Health Serv 2007;45(11):45–55.

72. Chafetz L, White M, Collins-Bride G, et al. Clinical trial of wellness training: health promotion for severely mentally ill adults. J Nerv Ment Dis 2008;196(6):475–83.

73. Lindenmayer JP, Khan A, Wance D, et al. Outcome evaluation of a structured educational wellness program in patient with severe mental illness. J Clin Psychiatry 2009;70(10):1385–96.

74. Van Citters AD, Pratt SI, Jue K, et al. A pilot evaluation of the In SHAPE individualized health promotion intervention for adults with mental illness. Community Ment Health J 2009. DOI: 10.1007/s10597-009-9297-x.

75. Druss BG, Zhao L, von Esenwein SA, et al. The Health and Recovery Peer (HARP) program: a peer-led intervention to improve medical self-management for persons with serious mental illness. Schizophr Res 2010;118:264–70.

76. Haupt DW, Rosenblatt LC, Kim E, et al. Prevalence and predictors of lipid and glucose monitoring in commercially insured patients treated with second-generation antipsychotic agents. Am J Psychiatry 2009;166(3):345–53.

77. Himelhoch S, Leith J, Goldberg R, et al. Care and management of cardiovascular risk factors among individuals with schizophrenia and type 2 diabetes who smoke. Gen Hosp Psychiatry 2009;31(1):30–2.

78. Kilbourne AM, Welsh D, McCarthy JF, et al. Quality of care for cardiovascular disease-related conditions in patients with and without mental disorders. J Gen Intern Med 2008;23(10):1628–33.

79. National Association of State Mental Health Program Directors, Medical Directors Council. Measurement of health status for people with serious mental illnesses. Alexandria (VA): National Association of State Mental Health Program Directors, Medical Directors Council; 2008.

80. Institute of Medicine. Improving the quality of health care for mental and substance-use conditions. Washington, DC: National Academies Press; 2006.

81. Coleman K, Austin BT, Brach C, et al. Evidence on the chronic care model in the new millennium. Health Aff 2009;28(1):75–85.

82. Everett A, Mahler J, Biblin J, et al. Improving the health of mental health consumers: effective policies and practices. Int J Ment Health 2008;37(2):8–48.

83. Buchanan RW, Kreyenbuhl J, Kelly DL, et al. The 2009 schizophrenia PORT psychopharmacological treatment recommendations and summary statements. Schizophr Bull 2010;36(1):71–93.

84. Marion LN, Braun S, Anderson D. Center for integrated health care: primary and mental health care for people with severe and persistent mental illnesses. J Nurs Educ 2004;43(2):71–4.

85. Sernyak MJ. Implementation of monitoring and management guidelines for second-generation antipsychotics. J Clin Psychiatry 2007;68(Suppl 4):14–8.

86. Lising-Enriquez K, George TP. Psychopharmacology for the clinician. J Psychiatry Neurosci 2009;34(3):E1–2.

87. American Diabetes Association, American Psychiatric Association, American Association of Clinical Endocrinologists, et al. Consensus development conference on antipsychotic drugs and obesity and diabetes. Diabetes Care 2004;27: 596–601.

88. Moore TA, Buchanan RW, Buckley PF, et al. The Texas medication algorithm project antipsychotic algorithm for schizophrenia: 2006 update. J Clin Psychiatry 2007;68(11):1751–62.

89. Brunero S, Lamont S, Fairbrother G. Prevalence and predictors of metabolic syndrome among patients attending an outpatient clozapine clinic in Australia. Arch Psychiatr Nurs 2009;23(3):261–8.

90. Marder SR, Essock SM, Miller AL, et al. Physical health monitoring of patients with schizophrenia. Am J Psychiatry 2004;161(8):1334–49.

91. Weiden PJ. Switching antipsychotics as a treatment strategy for antipsychotic-induced weight gain and dyslipidemia. J Clin Psychiatry 2007;68(Suppl 4):34–9.

92. Druss BG. Improving medical care for persons with serious mental illness: challenges and solutions. J Clin Psychiatry 2007;68(Suppl 4):40–4.

93. Gonder-Frederick LA, Cox DJ, Ritterband LM. Diabetes and behavioral medicine: the second decade. J Consult Clin Psychol 2002;70(3):611–25.

94. Dray-Spira R, Gary TL, Brancati FL. Socioeconomic position and cardiovascular disease in adults with and without diabetes: United States trends, 1997-2005. J Gen Intern Med 2008;23(10):1634–41.

95. Glazier RH, Bajcar J, Kennie NR, et al. A systematic review of interventions to improve diabetes care in socially disadvantaged populations. Diabetes Care 2006;29(7):1675–88.

96. Pignone M, DeWalt DA, Sheridan S, et al. Interventions to improve health outcomes for patients with low literacy: a systematic review. J Gen Intern Med 2005;20:185–92.

97. Kelly BD. Structural violence and schizophrenia. Soc Sci Med 2006;61:721–30.

98. Nordt C, Muller B, Rossler W, et al. Predictors and course of vocational status, income, and quality of life in people with severe mental illness: a naturalistic study. Soc Sci Med 2007;65(7):1420–9.

99. Hoffmann VP, Bushe C, Meyers AL, et al. A wellness program for patients with mental illness: self-reported outcomes. Prim Care Companion J Clin Psychiatry 2008;10(4):329–31.

100. Maj M. Physical illness and access to medical services in people with schizophrenia. Int J Ment Health 2008;37(1):13–21.

Resilience in Family Members of Persons with Serious Mental Illness

Jaclene A. Zauszniewski, PhD, RN-BC[a],*,
Abir K. Bekhet, PhD, RN, HSMI[b], M. Jane Suresky, DNP, PMHCNS-BC[a]

KEYWORDS

• Resilience • Family caregivers • Serious mental illness
• Risk/vulnerability factors • Positive/protective factors

The most recent census in the United States found that nearly 58 million adults had a diagnosed mental disorder[1] and 6% of these adults were diagnosed with a serious mental illness.[2] Before deinstitutionalization and advances in the development of medications, persons with serious mental illnesses lived in institutions, apart from their families. Today, these individuals live in our communities. Although some adults with mental illness live independently, many live with family members, who care for them and help them manage daily activities.[3,4] Even if they are not in the same household, family members are generally involved in their care and support.[5]

Family members of persons with serious mental illness may endure considerable stress and burden that can compromise their own health and quality of life and impair the functioning of the family. However, if family members are resilient, they can overcome stress associated with providing care for a loved one with a mental illness, and preserve their own health and the health of their family.[6,7] This integrative review summarizes current research on resilience in adult family members who have a relative with a serious mental disorder, including major depressive disorder, bipolar disorder, schizophrenia, and panic disorder.[8] Although some studies have included children and young siblings providing care for a relative with a mental illness, this review focuses on family members who are adults.

RESILIENCE

Early writings on resilience came from researchers who focused on its development in children and adolescents.[9,10] More recently, there has been an increased interest in

---

[a] Frances Payne Bolton School of Nursing, Case Western Reserve University, 10900 Euclid Avenue, Cleveland, OH 44106-4904, USA
[b] Marquette University College of Nursing, 530 North 16th Street, Milwaukee, WI 53233, USA
* Corresponding author.
E-mail address: jaz@case.edu

Nurs Clin N Am 45 (2010) 613–626
doi:10.1016/j.cnur.2010.06.007
0029-6465/10/$ – see front matter © 2010 Elsevier Inc. All rights reserved.
nursing.theclinics.com

resilience in adults[11] and families.[12] The concept of resilience was described by Rutter[13] as "relative resistance to psychosocial risk experiences" (p. 119), and by Luthar and colleagues[14] as "a dynamic process encompassing positive adaptation within the context of significant adversity." Richardson[15] defined resilience as "the process of coping with adversity, change, or opportunity in a manner that results in the identification, fortification, and enrichment of resilient qualities or protective factors" (p. 308). Definitions of resilience in caregivers vary,[16] but they all share the characteristic of overcoming adversity to not only survive the day-to-day burden of caring for a family member who is mentally ill, but to thrive; that is, to grow into a stronger, more flexible, and healthier person.[17] Resilience theory focuses on the strengths possessed by individuals or families that enable them to overcome adversity. The central constructs of resilience theory are risk or vulnerability factors, positive or protective factors, indicators of resilience, and outcomes of resilience.

RISK/VULNERABILITY FACTORS

Risk factors have been conceptualized as events or conditions associated with adversity, or factors that reduce one's ability to resist stressors or overcome adversity.[11] Vulnerability factors include traits, genetic predispositions, or environmental and biologic deficits. Potential risk factors in caring for a family member with a serious mental illness include caregiver strain, feelings of stigma, client dependence, and family disruption; together, these factors can seriously compromise the caregiver's resilience.[18] **Table 1** lists examples of risk or vulnerability factors that were identified in studies of family members of adults with serious mental illness.

Having a family member with a mental illness puts family members and the family unit at risk for experiencing negative outcome in terms of the physical and mental health of individual family members and the functioning of the family.[19,20] When the mentally ill family member is living in the same household, this may put relatives at greater risk for compromised health.[19,20] And the risk for poor health may increase even more when the mentally ill person requires ongoing supervision or direct personal care.[21] The lack of available, accessible, or affordable mental health services for

Table 1
Risk/vulnerability factors, protective factors, and outcomes of resilience indicators identified in studies of family members of adults with mental illness

Risk/Vulnerability Factors	Protective/Positive Factors	Outcomes of Resilience Indicators
Family member with mental illness	Control appraisal[24]	Expressed emotion[42]
Lack of mental health services/support	Positive appraisal[53]	Psychological well-being[19,24]
Threat appraisal[24]	Personal religiosity[22]	Family adaptation[48]
Caregiver age[22,23]	Psychoeducation[31–33]	Family functioning[49]
Education[23]	Social support[23]	Knowledge and understanding[21,59]
Caregiver burden/ stress[25–27]	Positive cognitions[18]	Morale[21]
Caregiver strain[27]	Length of time since diagnosis[34]	Relationship to mentally ill person[19]
Family disruption[27]	Age of care recipient[34]	Caregiver burden[23,28]
Stressful life events[28]		Quality of life[26,27]
Avoidance coping[25]		

families with a person with mental illness has been identified as a risk factor in several studies.[21]

Some demographic features of family caregivers may increase their vulnerability to compromised health, including age[22,23] and level of education.[23] The studies suggested that older family members and those who have less education may be more prone to health problems and disruptions in family functioning.

Family caregivers who appraise their situation as threatening are believed to be at greater risk.[24] They may perceive caregiving as burdensome or stressful,[25-27] and they report greater feelings of strain,[27] more stressful life events,[28] and greater disruption in family functioning.[27] Perlick and colleagues[25] found a high use of avoidance coping strategies by family members of persons with mental illness. Although avoidance coping may be a less-than-optimal method for coping, it is possible that this coping method may also be protective; thus, risk factors in one context may be protective in another.[11,13,29]

PROTECTIVE/POSITIVE FACTORS

According to Rutter,[30] protective factors reduce the effect of risk, decrease negative reactions to risk, promote resilience, and create opportunities for family caregivers, and include strategies for maintaining a positive success. Protective factors identified in studies of family members of adults with mental illness reflect their appraisal of the caregiving situation itself and their personal beliefs. A positive appraisal of the situation[24] and positive cognitions[18] have both been linked with greater resilience and better health outcomes. In addition, Murray-Swank and colleagues[22] found that personal religiosity helped family members of persons with mental illness adapt to the situation. Although positive appraisal, positive cognitions, and personal religiosity are intrapersonal factors that provide protection for family member of persons with mental illness, interpersonal and extrapersonal protective factors have also been identified.

Social support[23] and psychoeducation programs for family members[31-33] have been found to have positive effects on resilience and health outcomes for individuals and the family unit. Also, the duration of the caregiving experience, which is closely related to increasing age of the mentally ill care recipient, has been associated with resilience and quality of life in family members of adults with serious mental illness.[34]

RESILIENCE IN FAMILY CAREGIVERS

Only 3 studies of resilience in family members of persons with mental illness have been published, and all 3 were conducted more than a decade ago. Enns and colleagues[35] collected data on family resources, perceptions, and overall adaptation of 111 family members of adults admitted to a psychiatric hospital to identify factors that might contribute to resilience in family members. The data collected on major study variables were compared with averages on similar measures in the general population, and family members in the study were found to be similar to the general population on measures of health (p-norms = .546) and well-being (p-norms = .018), role performance (p-norms = .103), task accomplishment (p-norms = .424), and values and norms (p-norms = .308). They had significantly less perceived social support, esteem, and communication, and were less likely to seek spiritual support than the general population. However, they were more likely to acquire social support and to mobilize the immediate family, and they had higher scores on affective expression, communication, and perceived control.

Marsh and colleagues[36] conducted a national survey to investigate the effects of resilience among family members of people with mental illness. The 131 family members in the sample were mothers, fathers, wives, husbands, sisters, brothers, daughters, sons, and extended family members. Family members were asked to identify strengths within themselves, their family, or their mentally ill family member who they believed were developed in relation to their family member's mental illness. Personal resilience was reported most frequently (by 99% of participants), followed by family resilience (88%) and resilience in the mentally ill family member (76%). Mannion,[37] who did a follow-up analysis of the data from that survey, found that most spouses (83%) described a process of adaptation and recovery and cited personal resilience as a major factor in facilitating positive changes. Personal resilience was described more strongly than family resilience or resilience in the mentally ill family member.

These studies of resilience were all conducted in the 1990s. No recent studies have specifically examined resilience in family members of persons with serious mental illness. However, recent research has identified several strengths, characteristics, qualities, and virtues as indicators of resilience,[6,15,17] including acceptance, hardiness, hope, mastery, self-efficacy, sense of coherence, and resourcefulness. Studies that examined these resilience indicators in family members of persons with mental illness are reviewed later in this article.

Acceptance

Acceptance has been defined as a willingness to fully experience internal events, including thoughts, feelings, memories, and sensations.[38] It refers to an active process of understanding and having a sense of obligation and resignation to an unchangeable situation.[39] Christensen and Jacobson[40] defined acceptance as the ability to tolerate what might be regarded as an unpleasant behavior of a relative with mental illness, with some understanding of the deeper meaning of that behavior and an appreciation of its value and importance.

Four studies of family members of adults with mental illness have suggested that acceptance of the caregiving situation and the relative's diagnosis of mental illness is an indicator of resilience. In a study of 80 family members conducted in Ghana, Quinn[41] found that, in rural areas, families were more accepting of the mental illness and therefore more supportive of their loved ones. In a qualitative study conducted in Thailand, 17 Buddhist family members of persons with mental illness shared their beliefs and perspectives on their experiences with their mentally ill family member.[39] The themes they identified included management, compassion, and acceptance. Fortune and colleagues,[24] who examined relationships among perceptions of their loved one's psychosis, coping strategies, cognitive appraisals, and distress with 42 relatives of adults with schizophrenia, found that family members who expressed greater acceptance of their relative's psychosis, its severity, and consequences, experienced less distress ($r = -0.66$, $p<.001$). In addition, acceptance, along with positive reframing and a lower tendency toward self-blame, was found to mediate the effects of perceptions of their relative's illness on their distress.

Only 1 study has examined the needs of caregivers of people with mental illness in the United States. This intervention study by Eisner and Johnson[42] examined the effects of a psychoeducation program for 28 families who had a family member diagnosed with bipolar disorder. Their intervention also taught acceptance to the family members to decrease their anger and minimize self-blame. One week after the intervention, the family members were found to have more knowledge about their relative's illness, but their anger and self-blame remained unchanged. However, the results cannot be generalized because of the small sample size, and because baseline scores on criticism and anger were low. The study used self-report measures, and the length of the period was only 1 week, making it difficult to practice or implement what had been learned. Despite its limitations, this intervention study did address the needs of family members of persons with mental illness. Given the importance of the topic, more intervention studies are needed.

Hardiness

Hardiness was defined by Kobasa[43] as a personality characteristic consisting of 3 interrelated concepts: control, commitment, and challenge. However, others have said that hardiness involves cognitive and behavioral flexibility, motivation to follow through with plans, and endurance when faced with adversity.[44] In caregivers, hardiness has been found to minimize the burden of caregiving,[45] and enable caregivers to appraise the caregiving situation more positively,[46] and use problem-focused coping methods, including help-seeking strategies.[47]

Two studies have examined hardiness in family members of persons with mental illness. Greef and colleagues[48] studied 30 families of mentally ill young adults (average age 24 years) in Belgium, most of whom were diagnosed with schizophrenia or other psychosis or mood or anxiety disorder. Of 12 potential resilience indicators examined in that study, hardiness was found to have the strongest correlation with family adaptation ($r = 0.63$; $p<.01$). Also, Han and colleagues,[49] who collected data from 365 Korean families providing care for a relative with a chronic mental illness, found a significant correlation between hardiness and family functioning ($r = 0.51$, $p<.001$).

Neither of the 2 studies examined interventions; clearly intervention studies are needed to test the effects of programs to improve functioning in families with a relative with chronic mental illness. Large representative samples are also needed, as well as more focused homogeneous samples in terms of type of mental illness, length of illness, and age of the mentally ill person to be able to generalize the findings.

Mastery

Mastery has been defined as the extent to which individuals believe they have control over what happens in their life.[50] Thus, it can be conceptualized as a dimension of coping with stress that reflects a sense of personal control over potentially adverse circumstances. A sense of mastery has been identified as a resource that may facilitate family adaptation to mental illness.[51] In family caregivers, greater mastery has been associated with lower caregiver burden and psychological distress and a greater sense of competence in the caregiving role.[25,52]

Five studies of family members of persons with mental illness have examined mastery, which may be viewed as an indicator of resilience. Murray-Swank and colleagues[22] studied 83 caregivers of persons with serious mental illness to examine whether religiosity was associated with psychosocial adjustment and caregiver burden. The findings indicated that younger age and greater religiosity were both associated with mastery ($r = -0.28$, $p = .009$ and $r = 0.26$, $p = .017$).

Perlick and colleagues[25] studied 500 caregivers of adults with bipolar disorder to identify caregivers at risk for poor health in relation to caregiving and stress. The caregivers comprised 3 groups: those who were considered burdened, those considered effective, and those considered stigmatized. Those who were burdened experienced poorer health outcomes than the other 2 groups. They also reported lower mastery than the other groups ($F_{1,2} = 47.97$, $p<.001$).

Lau and Pang,[53] who examined how 129 relatives providing care for persons with major psychiatric illnesses appraised their caregiving, found that a better sense of mastery was associated with less negative appraisal ($r = -0.24, p = .03$); however, no relationship was found between mastery and positive appraisal of caregiving itself. Rose and colleagues[52] evaluated feelings of burden and sense of mastery of 30 family members of relatives with mental illness. No significant association was found between caregiver burden and mastery. The researchers explained that the lack of significance may have resulted from the mastery scale's inability to capture perceived lack of control among family members.

Pollio and colleagues[33] compared the effects of a psychoeducation group for 9 family members of adults with mental illness to usual services for family members. The 7 family members who completed the intervention showed significant improvements on 4 of 5 items measuring knowledge and mastery, and scores increased on the specific item that reflected feeling in control, although not significantly. Although these findings should be interpreted with caution, given the small sample, the results suggest that psychoeducation enhances a sense of mastery among family caregivers of persons with mental disorders. Future intervention research should use larger samples and analytical models with behavioral measures for both families and their ill members. Furthermore, outcomes should be measured immediately after the intervention, and 3 months, 6 months, and 1 year after the intervention to indicate whether mastery can be maintained over time.

Hope

Hope has been characterized as multidimensional and dynamic, with elements of confidence, but uncertain expectation of a positive outcome.[54] Hope is created from memories and influenced by relationships with others; it promotes forward movement and provides new insights and a sense of purpose.[55] Hope has been identified as an integral part of family members' ability to cope with mental illness in a family member.[56]

Seven studies have examined hope or optimism in family members of adults with mental illness. Bland and Darlington,[56] who conducted in-depth interviews with 16 family members in Australia to explore the meaning and importance of hope, found that hopefulness was an integral part of the coping process used by the family members. Karp and Tanarugsachock[57] conducted in-depth interviews with 50 family members of adults with depression, bipolar disorder, or schizophrenia to explore how family members managed their emotions during the course of the family member's mental illness. They found that it was at the point of diagnosis that feelings of hope were provoked in family members.

Using individual interviews and focus groups, Stjernswärd and Ostman[20] explored the experiences of 18 family members living with an individual with depression. The family members described hope as a motivating force for finding effective treatment, a trustworthy physician, a meaningful and productive future, and improved quality of life for both the mentally ill family member and themselves. Tweedell and colleagues[58] studied the experiences of 8 family members with a chronically mentally ill relative. During interviews conducted 5 times in a 1-year period, family members described hopes and fears associated with interpersonal relationships with their family member. They were unanimous in hoping their relatives would gain relief from suffering psychotic symptoms, return to their former selves, be independent in caring for themselves, and live a worthwhile and productive life. They also expressed cautious optimism that treatment would last, and some worried about losing hope for treatment, symptom management, and improved quality of life for their family member.

Pickett-Schenk and colleagues[21] studied 424 families of persons with schizophrenia who took part in an intervention designed to instill hope by providing education and support. Data were collected before the intervention and at 3 and 6 months following the program. At 3 months after the intervention, greater satisfaction with the education and support components of the intervention program predicted increased knowledge of the causes and treatment of mental illness ($\beta = 0.29$, $p<.001$ and $\beta = 0.21$, $p<.001$), greater understanding of mental health services ($\beta = 0.25$, $p<.001$ and $\beta = 0.34$, $p<.001$), and improved morale ($\beta = 0.19$, $p<.001$ and $\beta = 0.18$, $p<.001$). Some effects of satisfaction persisted at 6 months, but the effects on morale and understanding of mental heath services were not found 6 months after the intervention.

Pickett-Schenk and colleagues[19] also examined the effectiveness of the same intervention for 462 family members of adults with schizophrenia. As in the previous study, the intervention included education about the causes and treatment of mental illness, problem-solving and communication skills training, and family support. Outcomes were evaluated before intervention and at 3 and 6 months after the intervention. Family members in the intervention group reported better psychological well-being than those in a waiting list control group as indicated by fewer depressive symptoms ($\beta = -1.64$, $p = .04$), greater emotional role functioning ($\beta = 5.69$, $p = .03$) and vitality ($\beta = 3.57$, $p = .04$), and less negative views toward relationships with their mentally ill family member ($\beta = -0.73$, $p<.01$). These effects were maintained over time.

In a follow-up study, Pickett-Schenk and colleagues[59] examined the effects of the same intervention on family members' knowledge of causes and treatment of schizophrenia, problem-solving skills, and need for information. Those in the intervention group reported greater gains in knowledge than a waiting list control group ($\beta = 0.84$, $p<.01$), fewer needs for information on coping with positive and negative symptoms of their family member's illness ($\beta = -0.63$, $p<.05$ and $\beta = -0.80$, $p<.001$, respectively), and greater gains in problem management ($\beta = -1.00$, $p<.001$), basic facts about mental illness and its treatment ($\beta = -0.73$, $p<.01$), and community resources ($\beta = -0.07$, $p<.05$). The effects were maintained over time.

Of these 7 studies, only 1 was a randomized controlled trial[19] and the randomized controlled trial had some limitations, including a possible placebo effect and use of self-reported data, making it difficult to determine whether the intervention brought about actual improvements in the family members' relationships with their mentally ill relatives.[19] Intervention studies that include behavioral observations rather than self-report are needed.

Self-Efficacy

Self-efficacy refers to an individual's confidence in dealing with challenging and stressful encounters,[60] or the self-evaluation of one's capacity for performing an activity or task to achieve a specific goal.[61] In family caregivers of persons with mental illness, greater self-efficacy has been linked with better management of behavioral problems in care receivers, less perceived stress, and lower subjective burden.[6]

Two studies have examined self-efficacy of family members of adults with schizophrenia. Both studies involved Chinese family members. Cheng and Chan[32] evaluated the effectiveness of a psychoeducation program with 64 family caregivers recruited from a mental hospital in Hong Kong. Those in the psychoeducation group improved more in self-efficacy than a group receiving routine care ($t = -7.16$, $p<.01$). The effectiveness of the psychoeducation program was then tested in another study of 73 Chinese family caregivers of persons with schizophrenia[31]; this study also examined longer-term effects. Postintervention effects on self-efficacy were similar to those in the first study and these effects were sustained at 6 months, but not at 12 months, indicating a need for continued intervention to promote self-efficacy.

Although both studies provided promising results, they had several limitations. For example, the measures used were self-reported, and the mentally ill persons were primarily men, although caregivers were women.[31] Also, the studies included only family members who were willing to participate, so this group might have had more motivation to change, leading to positive outcomes.[32]

Sense of Coherence

A sense of coherence has been defined as a global orientation toward life that involves cognitive, behavioral, and motivational elements, and is expressed in the belief that the world is comprehensible, manageable, and meaningful.[62] Family sense of coherence refers to the belief of family members that the internal and external environments are structured and predictable and that resources are available; they perceive life and their situation as a meaningful challenge and consider that they can exert an influence on the course of events.[48]

Five studies have evaluated sense of coherence in family members of adults with mental illness. Han and colleagues,[49] who examined the influence of a sense of coherence on family functioning in 365 Korean families providing care for a relative with a chronic mental illness, found a significant positive correlation between sense of coherence and family functioning ($r = 0.43$; $p<.001$). Greef and colleagues[48] examined sense of coherence as an indicator of adaptation in 30 families of mentally ill persons in Belgium. Hardiness showed the strongest correlation with sense of coherence ($r = 0.63$; $p<.01$). In a study of 556 Thai family caregivers of adults with schizophrenia, Pipatananond and colleagues[23] found that sense of coherence was influenced by education ($\gamma = 0.29$, $p<.001$), income ($\gamma = 0.28$, $p<.001$), social support ($\gamma = 0.20$, $p<.001$), and perceived seriousness of illness ($\gamma = 0.23$, $p<.001$), and sense of coherence had a direct negative effect on caregiver burden ($\beta = 0.16$, $p<.001$).[23]

In a study of 60 American women who were family members of adults with serious mental illness, Suresky and colleagues[26] found that caregiver burden had a negative effect on sense of coherence ($\beta = -0.33$; $p<.01$), although sense of coherence accounted for 41% of the variance in quality of life and partially mediated the effects of caregiver burden on quality of life.[26] In a follow-up study on the same women, Zauszniewski and colleagues[18] found that the effects of caregiver burden on sense of coherence were mediated by positive cognitions, which served as protective factors.

No studies have evaluated interventions for sense of coherence in family members of adults with mental illness, and the studies reviewed had some limitations. Most were either cross-sectional[23,48,49] or secondary analyses[18,26] and, therefore, it is difficult to assess changes in study variables over time. Convenience sampling limits the generalizability of the findings, and the samples were heterogeneous in type of mental illness, length of illness, single parent or intact family, and age of the mentally ill family member.[48] Also, given the small samples, caution must be used in drawing conclusions from the findings.[18,26,48]

Resourcefulness

Resourcefulness may be defined as cognitive and behavioral skills that are used to prevent potentially negative effects of thoughts, feelings, or sensations on the performance of daily activities[63] and to obtain assistance from others when unable to function independently.[64] Personal and social resourcefulness skills are complementary, can fluctuate over time, and are equally important for optimal quality of life.[65]

Four studies have examined resourcefulness in family caregivers of persons with serious mental illness. Wang and colleagues[28] examined the effects of resourcefulness on stressful life events, psychiatric care activities, and the burden faced by 81 family caregivers of schizophrenic adolescents. The study found that 24.5% of the variance ($F_{5,75}$ = 6.20, p<.001) in caregiver burden was explained by psychiatric care activities and the interaction of stressful life events and resourcefulness, indicating that resourcefulness moderated the adverse effects of stressful life events on caregiver burden.

Zauszniewski and colleagues[34] studied 60 women who were family members of adults diagnosed with schizophrenia, bipolar disorder, depression, or a panic anxiety disorder to identify factors that might affect family members' resourcefulness. Increasing age of the mentally ill person and longer time since diagnosis were associated with greater personal resourcefulness (r = 0.32, p<.01 and r = 0.35, p<.01, respectively). The women who were caregivers of adults with schizophrenia had greater personal and resourcefulness ($t_{1,52}$ = 4.19, p<.01 and $t_{1,52}$ = 2.62, p<.01, respectively) than women who had a family member with bipolar disorder. Sisters of mentally ill persons reported more social resourcefulness than did mothers, daughters, or wives ($F_{2,59}$ = −3.16, p<.05), but there were no significant differences in personal resourcefulness.

In a follow-up study of the same women, Zauszniewski and colleagues[27] found that African American and white women reported similar resourcefulness skills. However, in African Americans, greater caregiver burden was associated with lower resourcefulness (r = −0.38, p<.0010) and lower resourcefulness correlated with poorer mental health (r = 0.53, p<.001), suggesting that resourcefulness may mediate the adverse effects of caregiver burden on mental health. Another follow-up study by Zauszniewski and colleagues[18] focused on the mediating role played by positive cognitions, conceptualized as a protective factor, on the relationship between caregiver burden and resourcefulness. The findings from that study provide support for resilience theory in that positive cognitions mediated the effects of caregiver burden on resourcefulness, an indicator of resilience.

All 4 of these studies were cross-sectional or secondary analyses, and none included an intervention. The studies also had some limitations, such as convenience samples, cross-sectional design, and small sample sizes.[18,27,34] Longitudinal studies of larger and more diverse samples of family members of mentally ill persons, including men and persons from racial/ethnic minorities, are recommended. Intervention studies that teach cognitive behavioral self-help and help-seeking skills are also needed. Addressing the needs of family members of adolescents with serious mental illness is important; thus, intervention studies are needed for this vulnerable population.

OUTCOMES OF RESILIENCE

Resilience and resilience indicators have been linked with several positive health outcomes for individuals and families.[17] In the studies of family members of adults with mental illness included in this review, resilience indicators were found to be associated with and, in some cases, to affect or predict outcomes that indicate mental and physical health and quality of life in individual family members and optimal family functioning.

On the individual level, resilience indicators have been linked with decreased caregiver burden in family members of persons with mental illness.[23,28] In addition, decreased levels of expressed emotion, defined as a critical, hostile, or overinvolved attitude toward a relative with mental illness, have been associated with greater resilience in family members of persons with mental illness.[42] Other outcomes of resilience indicators found in studies of family members include better morale,[21] greater psychological well-being,[19,24] and improved knowledge and understanding of their family member's diagnosis.[21,59] Two studies of family members found that enhanced quality of life was associated with indicators of resilience.[26,27] Greater resilience may also be linked with improvement in family members' relationships with their relative with a psychiatric diagnosis.[19] Resilience has also been associated with greater family adaptation[48] and improvement in family functioning.[49]

SUMMARY

Although resilience has been examined in studies of family caregivers, few studies have included family members of persons with serious mental illness. However, many researchers have examined characteristics of family members of persons with mental illness that may be considered indicators of resilience, including acceptance, hardiness, hope, mastery, self-efficacy, sense of coherence, and resourcefulness. The research has consistently shown that family members who possess these positive characteristics are better able to manage and overcome adversity associated with caring for a family member diagnosed with a mental illness. Thus, enhancement of the resilience of family members of persons with serious mental illness contributes to both their own well-being and the well-being of those for whom they provide care.

The findings from the studies reviewed here provide beginning evidence of the importance of focusing nursing interventions on supporting and enhancing the resilience of family members of individuals with mental illness. However, additional studies to develop and test interventions for enhancing the characteristics constituting resilience in these family members are needed. Longitudinal studies that measure outcomes immediately after the intervention and at 3 months, 6 months, and 1 year after the intervention would provide a picture of how resilience indicators can be enhanced and maintained. Also, intervention studies that include behavioral observation, rather than relying solely on self-report, are needed. The evidence that emerges from testing well-developed interventions can inform clinical practice and enrich psychiatric nurses' ability to provide quality care for patients and their families.

Advanced practice nurses (APNs) need to take a focused family therapy approach to manage stress and disruption in the family environment, to build the family's resilience and contribute to improvement in quality of life for the family and the person who is mentally ill. Assessing family members' level of hardiness, sense of coherence, hope, and resourcefulness using standardized measures at the start of a treatment plan for family therapy could provide baseline data and direction for therapy. Assisting the family to gain knowledge of the mental illness and associated behaviors would facilitate understanding of the patient's situation. In addition to using a cognitive approach to therapy, APNs might suggest adjunct therapies for individual family members. For example, yoga has been found to be beneficial in reducing anxiety and depression, acupuncture is used to treat stress, and self-hypnosis provides a feeling of letting go of internal pressure and discomfort. At the conclusion of therapy, hardiness, sense of coherence, hope, and resourcefulness should be measured again and compared with baseline results to provide further direction for therapy.

The information derived from the current review can be used by psychiatric nurses to plan primary, secondary, and tertiary prevention strategies to help caregivers of persons with mental illness regain, attain, or maintain optimal wellness. Assessing an individual's attitude toward mental illness, and his or her strengths and concerns, is vital to facilitate adjustment. Secondary prevention should be implemented when stress symptoms have already developed. Secondary prevention should encompass interventions to increase resilience for those with stress as a result of their caregiving. Tertiary prevention would help caregivers to use all existing internal and external resources to prevent further stress and maintain optimal wellness.

REFERENCES

1. US Census Bureau. Population estimates by demographic characteristics. Table 2: annual estimates of the population by selected age groups and sex for the United States: April 1, 2000 to July 1, 2004. US Census Bureau: Population Division 2005 (NC-EST2004–02).
2. Kessler RC, Chiu WT, Demler O, et al. Prevalence, severity, and comorbidity of 12-month DSM-IV disorders in the National Comorbidity Survey replication. Arch Gen Psychiatry 2005;62:617–27.
3. Kohn-Wood LP, Wilson MN. The context of caretaking in rural areas: family factors influencing the level of functioning of seriously mentally ill patients living at home. Am J Community Psychol 2005;36(1/2):1–13.
4. Wynaden D, Ladzinski U, Lapsley J, et al. The caregiving experience: how much do health professionals understand? Collegian 2006;13(3):6–10.
5. Lively S, Friedrich RM, Rubenstein L. The effect of disturbing illness behaviors on siblings of persons with schizophrenia. J Am Psychiatr Nurses Assoc 2004;10(5): 222–32.
6. Saunders JC. Families living with severe mental illness: a literature review. Issues Ment Health Nurs 2003;24(2):175–98.
7. Walton-Moss B, Gerson L, Rose L. Effects of mental illness on family quality of life. Issues Ment Health Nurs 2005;26:627–42.
8. Bye L, Partridge J. State level classification of serious mental illness: a case for a more uniform standard. J Health Soc Policy 2004;19(2):1–29.
9. Garmezy N, Rutter M. Stress, coping, and development in children. New York: McGraw-Hill; 1983.
10. Werner EE, Smith RS. Overcoming the odds: high risk children from birth to adulthood. Ithaca (NY): Cornell University Press; 1992.
11. Smith-Osborne A. Life span and resiliency theory: a critical review. Adv Soc Work 2007;18(1):152–68.
12. McCubbin MA, McCubbin HI. Resiliency in families: a conceptual model of family adjustment and adaptation in response to stress and crises. In: McCubbin HI, Thompson AI, McCubbin MA, editors. Family assessment: resiliency, coping, and adaptation—Inventories for research and practice. Madison (WI): University of Wisconsin System; 1996. p. 1–64.
13. Rutter M. Resilience concepts and findings: implications for family therapy. J Fam Ther 1999;2:119–44.
14. Luthar S, Cicchetti D, Becker B. The construct of resilience: a critical evaluation and guidelines for future work. Child Dev 2000;71:543–62.
15. Richardson GE. The metatheory of resilience and resiliency. J Clin Psychol 2002; 58(3):307–21.
16. Gillespie BM, Chaboyer W, Wallis M. Development of a theoretically derived model of resilience through concept analysis. Contemp Nurse 2007;25(1/2):124–35.
17. Van Breda AD. Resilience theory: a literature review. Pretoria (South Africa): South African Military Health Service; 2001.
18. Zauszniewski JA, Bekhet AK, Suresky MJ. Effects on resilience of women family caregivers of adults with serious mental illness: the role of positive cognitions. Arch Psychiatr Nurs 2009;23(6):412–22.

19. Pickett-Schenk SA, Cook JA, Steigman P, et al. Psychological well-being and relationship outcomes in a randomized study of family-led education. Arch Gen Psychiatry 2006;63:1043–50.

20. Stjernswärd S, Ostman M. Whose life am I living? Relatives living in the shadow of depression. Int J Soc Psychiatry 2008;54(4):358–69.

21. Pickett-Schenk SA, Cook JA, Laris A. Journey of Hope program outcomes. Community Ment Health J 2000;36:413–24.

22. Murray-Swank AB, Lucksted A, Medoff DR, et al. Religiosity, psychosocial adjustment, and subjective burden of persons who care for those with mental illness. Psychiatr Serv 2006;57(3):361–5.

23. Pipatananond P, Boontong T, Hanucharurnkul S, et al. Caregiver burden predictive model: an empirical test among caregivers for the schizophrenic. Thai J Nurs Res 2006;6(2):24–40.

24. Fortune DG, Smith JV, Garvey K. Perceptions of psychosis, coping, appraisals, and psychological distress in the relatives of patients with schizophrenia: an exploration using self-regulation theory. Br J Clin Psychol 2005;44:319–31.

25. Perlick DA, Rosenheck RA, Miklowitz DJ, et al. Caregiver burden and health in bipolar disorder: a cluster analytic approach. J Nerv Ment Dis 2008;196(6):484–91.

26. Suresky MJ, Zauszniewski JA, Bekhet AK. Sense of coherence and quality of life in women family members of the seriously mentally ill. Issues Ment Health Nurs 2008;29:265–78.

27. Zauszniewski JA, Bekhet AK, Suresky MJ. Relationships among stress, depressive cognitions, resourcefulness and quality of life in female relatives of seriously mentally ill adults. Issues Ment Health Nurs 2009;30:142–50.

28. Wang S, Rong J, Chen C, et al. [A study of stress, learned resourcefulness and caregiver burden among primary caregivers of schizophrenic adolescents]. J Nurs 2007;54(5):37–47 [in Chinese].

29. Ungar M. A constructionist discourse on resilience: multiple contexts, multiple realities among at-risk children and youth. Youth Soc 2004;35(3):341–65.

30. Rutter M. Psychosocial resilience and protective mechanisms. Am J Orthopsychiatry 1987;57:316–31.

31. Chan SW, Yip B, Tso S, et al. Evaluation of a psychoeducation program from Chinese clients with schizophrenia and their family caregivers. Patient Educ Couns 2009;75:67–76.

32. Cheng LY, Chan SW. Psychoeducation program for Chinese family carers of members with schizophrenia. West J Nurs Res 2005;27(5):583–99.

33. Pollio DE, North CS, Osborne VA. Family-responsive psychoeducation groups for families with an adult member with mental illness: pilot results. Community Ment Health J 2002;38(5):413–21.

34. Zauszniewski JA, Bekhet AK, Suresky MJ. Factors associated with perceived burden, resourcefulness, and quality of life in female family members of adults with serious mental illness. J Am Psychiatr Nurses Assoc 2008;14(2):125–35.

35. Enns R, Reddon J, McDonald L. Indications of resilience among family members of people admitted to a psychiatric facility. Psychiatr Rehabil J 1999;23(2):127–33.

36. Marsh DT, Lefley HP, Evans-Rhodes D, et al. The family experience of mental illness: evidence for resilience. Psychiatr Rehabil J 1996;20(2):3–12.

37. Mannion E. Resilience and burden in spouses of people with mental illness. Psychiatr Rehabil J 1996;20(2):13–23.

38. Orsillo SM, Roemer L, Block-Lerner J, et al. Acceptance, mindfulness, and cognitive-behavioral therapy: comparisons, contrasts and applications to

anxiety. In: Hayes SC, Follette VM, Linehan MM, editors. Mindfulness and acceptance: expanding the cognitive-behavioral tradition. New York: Guilford Press; 2004. p. 66–95.

39. Sethabouppha H, Kane C. Caring for the seriously mentally ill in Thailand: Buddhist family caregiving. Arch Psychiatr Nurs 2005;19(2):44–57.
40. Christensen A, Jacobson NS. Reconcilable differences. New York: Guilford Press; 2000.
41. Quinn N. Beliefs and community responses to mental illness in Ghana: the experiences of family carers. Int J Soc Psychiatry 2007;53(2):175–88.
42. Eisner LR, Johnson SL. An acceptance-based psychoeducation intervention to reduce expressed emotion in relatives of bipolar patients. Behav Ther 2008;39: 375–85.
43. Kobasa SC. Stressful life events, personality and health: an inquiry into hardiness. J Pers Soc Psychol 1979;37:1–11.
44. Maddi SR. On hardiness and other pathways to resilience. Am Psychol 2005; 60(3):261–2.
45. DiBartolo M. Exploring self-efficacy and hardiness in spousal caregivers of individuals with dementia. J Gerontol Nurs 2002;28(4):24–33.
46. DiBartolo M, Soeken K. Appraisal, coping, hardiness, and self-perceived health in community-dwelling spouse caregivers of persons with dementia. Res Nurs Health 2003;26(6):445–58.
47. Clark P. Effects of individual and family hardiness on caregiver depression and fatigue. Res Nurs Health 2002;25(1):37–48.
48. Greef AP, Vansteenwegen A, Ide M. Resiliency in families with a member with a psychological disorder. Am J Fam Ther 2006;34:285–300.
49. Han K, Lee P, Park E, et al. Family functioning and mental illness: a Korean correlational study. Asian J Nurs 2007;10(2):129–36.
50. Pearlin LI, Schooler C. The structure of coping. J Health Soc Behav 1978;19: 2–21.
51. Rungreangkulkij S, Gillis CL. Conceptual approached to studying family caregiving for persons with severe mental illness. J Fam Nurs 2000;6(4):341–66.
52. Rose LE, Mallinson RK, Gerson LD. Mastery, burden, and areas of concern among family caregivers of mentally ill persons. Arch Psychiatr Nurs 2006; 20(1):41–51.
53. Lau D, Pang A. Caregiving experience for Chinese caregivers of persons suffering from severe mental disorders. Hong Kong J Psychiatr 2007;17:75–80.
54. Dufault K, Martocchio B. Hope: its spheres and dimensions. Nurs Clin North Am 1985;20(2):379–91.
55. Parse RR. Hope: an international human becoming perspective. Boston: Jones and Hartlett; 2000.
56. Bland R, Darlington Y. The nature and sources of hope: perspectives of family caregivers of people with serious mental illness. Perspect Psychiatr Care 2002; 38(2):61–8.
57. Karp DA, Tanarugsachock V. Mental illness, caregiving, and emotional management. Qual Health Res 2000;10(1):6–25.
58. Tweedell D, Forchuk C, Jewell J, et al. Families' experience during recovery or nonrecovery from psychosis. Arch Psychiatr Nurs 2004;18(1):17–25.
59. Pickett-Schenk SA, Lippincott RC, Bennett C, et al. Improving knowledge about mental illness through family-led education: the journey of hope. Psychiatr Serv 2008;59(1):49–56.
60. Bandura A. Self-efficacy: the exercise of control. New York: WH Freeman; 1997.

61. Zulkosky K. Self-efficacy: a concept analysis. Nurs Forum 2009;44(2):93–102.
62. Antonovsky A. Health, stress, and coping. San Francisco (CA): Jossey-Bass; 1979.
63. Rosenbaum M. Learned resourcefulness on coping skills, self-control, and adaptive behavior. New York: Springer; 1990.
64. Nadler A. Help-seeking behavior as a coping resource. In: Rosenbaum M, editor. Learned resourcefulness: on coping skills, self-control, and adaptive behavior. New York: Springer; 1990. p. 127–64.
65. Zauszniewski JA. Resourcefulness. In: Fitzpatrick JJ, Wallace M, editors. Encyclopedia of nursing research. New York: Springer; 2006. p. 526–8.

Policy Issues in Mental Health Among the Elderly

Karen M. Robinson, PhD, PMHCNS-BC

KEYWORDS

• Policy issues • Mental disorders • Elders

Americans are living longer than ever before in history. The Centers for Disease Control and Prevention (CDC)[1] predicts that the number of persons older than 65 years will increase from approximately 35 million in 2000 to an estimated 71 million in 2030, comprising approximately 20% of the US population. The CDC[1] further estimates that the number of persons older than 80 years is expected to increase from 9.3 million in 2000 to 19.5 million in 2030. With age comes an increased risk for chronic mental health disorders. About 1 in 8 baby boomers is expected to be diagnosed with Alzheimer disease, which will amount to some 10 million members of this age cohort.[2] Dementia tends to be the mental disorder most often associated with old age.[3] The debilitating nature of this disease and the intensity of care required guarantee that a particularly heavy demand will be placed on the US health care system. Age is the largest risk factor, with 49% of the population older than 85 years diagnosed with dementia.[2]

The prevalence of mental health disorders among the elderly is often unrecognized. One in four older adults lives with depression, anxiety disorders, or other significant psychiatric disorders.[4] Mental health disorders are frequently comorbid in older adults, occurring with a number of common chronic illnesses such as in diabetes, cardiac disease, and arthritis.[5] Functional declines are more pronounced in comorbid mental and physical disorders, thus threatening the elderly's abilities and capacity for self care. A spiral relationship evolves over time as a mental health disorder (such as depression or anxiety) and increases risk for self-perceived functional and behavioral disabilities. For example, a coexisting cognitive disorder such as Alzheimer disease co-occurring with diabetes threatens the person's ability to understand how to manage blood glucose measurement and readings, thus further eroding self-care management of diabetes.[5] The public is becoming more aware of the aging of the population and the difficulties that are exacerbated by unmet services and limited access to mental health services. This article describes policy issues related to chronic mental health disorders and the older population. Mental health parity, a recent

School of Nursing, University of Louisville, 555 South Floyd Street, Louisville, KY 40292, USA
E-mail address: Kmrobi01@louisville.edu

Nurs Clin N Am 45 (2010) 627–634
doi:10.1016/j.cnur.2010.06.005
0029-6465/10/$ – see front matter © 2010 Elsevier Inc. All rights reserved.

nursing.theclinics.com

policy issue occurring at the national level, is discussed first followed by workforce issues specific to the discipline of nursing.

MENTAL HEALTH PARITY: A NATIONAL POLICY ISSUE

Historically, the perception of the public about mental illness differed from other physical illnesses because of the stigma related to mental illness. The perception held by the public was that society needed protection from people with mental illness by providing care in isolated institutions on the outskirts of town.[6] Mental health care evolved during the years from prisonlike conditions to many forms of treatment financed by state mental health systems. Institutionalization of the most seriously ill propagated the myth that mental illness was "incurable" despite many advances in treatment.[6(p.77)] This negative perception and stigma make mental health parity laws difficult for the public to support. When parity laws are in place, health plans operating in the private health insurance market are required to provide an equivalent level of coverage for the treatment of mental health disorders that is provided for physical disorders. The passage of recent federal mental health parity legislation sent a strong message that mental health disorders are just as treatable as other physical disorders.[7]

Advocacy for Mental Health Parity

At the national level, mental health parity has been proposed since President John F. Kennedy directed the first attempt to regulate insurance coverage for mental health through the US Civil Services, the predecessor agency to the US Office of Personnel Management. Mental health parity was first offered in 2 nationally available Federal Employee Health Benefits (FEHB) Program health plans, Blue Cross Blue Shield and Aetna.[8]

Appeals for parity were framed in many different ways during the political debate. Parity can be framed as a response to market failure, as an antidiscrimination measure, or as a strategy to improve equity and alleviate the financial burden of mental illness.[9] Current success in passage of parity laws resulted primarily because of focus on all 3 arguments.

The debate began historically with the fairness argument that insurance should not discriminate against individuals with mental illness. To investigate this argument, Busch and Barry[10] examined whether state parity laws differentially affected the use of services among people with low income or those with poor mental health. Findings indicated that persons in smaller employee firms were more likely to use services after the implementation of parity and that this effect was concentrated among people with low income. Before the implementation of parity, people with low income were not able to access mental health services. Thus, parity can be viewed as a way to prevent discrimination against people with low income who have a mental disorder.

Another fear about passage of a mental health parity law was that equivalence would dramatically increase costs for employers and drive up premiums for patients or result in claims for frivolous services. These fears have not materialized even with broad parity laws in place.[11] The experience across more than 45 states that have passed parity laws and of the federal government (parity has been provided under the FEHB program since 2001) is that parity does not substantially increase utilization or cost.[7,10] Evidence from the FEHB program, which provided equal coverage for specialty mental health and substance abuse services for 8 million members in 2001, suggested achievement of a real cost saving in the amount of $40 on average annually per treatment user.[12] Even large businesses have recognized the value of including mental health parity in their insurance packages. Mental health and substance abuse account for more disability than any other health condition, and 217 million days of work are lost annually because of disability related to mental illness and substance abuse disorders, costing US employers $17 billion per year. The effect of parity on disability, return to work, and absenteeism was measured, and parity was determined to be cost effective. A landmark report by the National Business Group on Health recommended employers equalize their medical and behavioral health benefit given evidence that parity yields significant clinical benefits without increasing overall health care costs.[7]

Mental Health Parity Legislation

Two important changes in health insurance coverage for mental health and substance abuse disorders were enacted into law in 2008 and will take effect in 2010. The goal of a nationwide push for mental health parity was to provide equal coverage for mental disorders on par with physical disorders. The Paul Wellstone and Pete Domenici Mental Health Parity and Addiction Equity Act of 2008, signed into law on October 3, 2008, does not mandate coverage. Rather, the legislation affects large employers. Medicaid managed care plans, and some State Children's Health Insurance Program plans offered group health insurance with mental health or substance abuse coverage. Another less-known parity law was also enacted in 2008 when the Congress enacted the Medicare Improvements for Patients and Providers Act, which phases in mental health parity for Medicare recipients. These 2 laws supplement mental health parity legislation now in force in every state except Idaho and Wyoming.[13]

Wellstone-Domenici Act

This parity legislation applies to any organization with 50 or more employees and includes self-funded plans. More than half of the employer-sponsored plans were self-funded and were previously not subject to state mental health parity laws. One of the most important accomplishments of the 2008 Wellstone-Domenici Act is that new financial protections are offered to the most severely ill persons who need intensive mental health treatment and inpatient care. For example, before this legislation, adults with bipolar disorder or schizophrenia might spend $15,000 to $20,000 in medical bills per year for inpatient stays and other intensive treatment, most of which now are covered under the new law. The law also eliminates arbitrary limits on outpatient visits, translating into fewer out-of-pocket expenses for those who see a therapist or addiction counselor on a continuing basis.[11,13]

Medicare Mental Health Parity

The law authorizing mental health parity for Medicare recipients will be phased in over several years. Medicare enrolls people who are 65 years of age and older as well as younger people who are permanently disabled. Currently, Medicare recipients must pay half of the cost for outpatient psychotherapy and other mental health services. Starting in 2010, the copay will be reduced gradually until it reaches 20% in 2014, which is equivalent to the current Medicare copay for other outpatient health services. Another feature of the Medicare parity law provided for expanded coverage of prescription antidepressants, antipsychotics, and anticonvulsants.[13] After passage of the parity legislation requiring coverage for mental health services, Trivedi and colleagues[14] wondered whether the use of timely follow-up care would increase after a psychiatric hospitalization. Researchers explored the relationship between mental health parity and use of timely follow-up care after a psychiatric hospitalization. Seniors (N = 43,892) enrolled in 173 group health plans and Medicare Part B who had been hospitalized for a mental illness were tracked regarding their follow-up mental health visits within 7 to 30 days following a psychiatric hospitalization. Indeed, Medicare enrollees in plans with mental health parity had a markedly greater use of clinically appropriate mental health services following a hospitalization.[14] Because of increased follow up after a psychiatric hospitalization, parity may reduce the revolving door cycle that follows many psychiatric hospitalizations.

INCREASING ACCESS TO MENTAL HEALTH SERVICES

With the passage of mental health parity legislation plus the possibility of future health reform with resulting changes in the health care system, the demand for increased access to mental health services presents exciting opportunities focusing attention on areas that have historically been underrepresented and underresourced. One such underresourced area is the future mental health care workforce. In its seminal report, *Retooling for an Aging America*, the Institute of Medicine (IOM)[15] documents 3 critical points that indicate that the time to act is now: (1) nurses make up the largest population of the health care workforce, (2) most nurses are at some point involved in the care of the elderly, and (3) basic educational curriculums for Registered Nurses (RNs) include little preparation in principles for geriatric or geropsychiatric nursing (GPN). Thus, most of the nursing workforce is unprepared to meet the needs of elders living with mental disorders.

Workforce for an Aging America

According to the IOM report, the bottom line for projected workforce needs in 2030 (assuming that current patterns of care continue) is that America will need 3.5 million more health care workers for older Americans. This projection includes an anticipated need for 868,000 more RNs and 231,000 more licensed practical and vocational nurses. This will be a tall order to fill given that the nation today already has an estimated 118,000 currently unfilled nursing positions in hospital settings alone. A shortage of 500,000 nurses is projected to occur by 2025. Buerhaus,[16] taking note of the aging of the nursing workforce, has considerable doubt about the nation's ability to furnish the needed supply because there are "no good substitutes for nurses".[(p.38)] The demand for nurses will continue to increase in the next 7 to 9 years.

Aging of the Psychiatric-Mental Health Nurse Workforce in the United States

Since 1975, the Health Resources and Services Administration has completed surveys assessing the supply, composition, and distribution of RNs at state and national levels. Hanrahan[17] used the 2004 National Sample Survey of Registered Nurses[18] to examine the Psychiatric-Mental Health RN (PMH RN) population in the United States. RN survey respondents who answered the question "What type of patient is primarily treated in the unit/organization in which you work?" with "psychiatric" were included as the PMH RN sample. The total estimated number of PMH RNs in the United States was 90,765.[18] Nonpsychiatric nurses (N = 2,818,592) and PMH RNs (N = 90,765) were compared to determine unique characteristics of psychiatric nurses. The typical profile of a PMH RN (according to Hanrahan[17]) was a 50-year-old woman (aged 56 years in 2009) who was married, white, and living in an urban setting. The typical PMH RN has more than 26 years of experience and most likely works full time in either a hospital or a community health care setting performing direct patient care with supervisory functions. She identifies having a 20% chance of leaving her position, primarily because of burnout or stress. Odds are at 52% that she has attained a baccalaureate or master's degree in nursing. Average annual salary for a full-time PMH RN position was identified at $57,450 in 2004.[17]

Psychiatric nursing attracts nearly twice as many men (10.2%) when compared with nonpsychiatric nursing (5.6%). The number of men, however, is still very small. The atypical PMH RN is a 40-year-old man who is married, white, and living in an urban area and has 11 to 15 years of experience and working full time in a hospital or community health care setting performing direct patient care and supervision. He is less likely to teach, consult, or work in a long-term care setting but is more likely to be an administrator than the typical PMH RN. He has attained an educational level of an associate degree in nursing but is likely to have a baccalaureate or higher degree in another field. Average annual salary for his full-time PMH RN position was $62,912 in 2004. Thus, men in psychiatric nursing receive higher salaries and fill more administrative positions. But gender disparity issues, apparent in other disciplines, also pervade psychiatric nursing.[17]

When comparing psychiatric nurses with nonpsychiatric nurses, on average the psychiatric nurse at mean age of 50 years was 3.6 years older than the nonpsychiatric nurse at mean age of 46.7 years. Only 4.2% of the psychiatric nurses were younger than 30 years, compared with 9% of nonpsychiatric nurses. Of significance was the fact that more psychiatric nurses were aged 50 years or older (59%) compared with nonpsychiatric nurses (41%). Assuming the retirement age is 66 years, more than half of the current psychiatric nurse workforce may leave their jobs by 2018. Because more than two-thirds of PMH RNs work in hospitals and have an average of 26 years of experience, one of the first settings that retirement will hit the hardest will be hospitals where psychiatric nurses work. Psychiatric inpatient settings today have become far more complex, uncertain, and volatile. The unit census is almost always filled with seriously ill patients.[19] One of the most important roles of a PMH RN is keeping the environment safe for patients and staff.[20] Within 10 years, nearly half of the current PMH RN workforce may have retired. In addition, data indicate that one-quarter of nurses leave their positions each year.[17] Combined, the loss of experienced and retired PMH RNs from the hospital workforce may have devastating effects on a system already maximally stretched.[19]

More than just the hospital inpatient care will be affected by the aging of the PMH RN workforce. Community-based care will be needed more than ever, with mental health parity providing for increased access to care. Likewise, home and community-based services, including monitoring and managing mental health care in the home, will be needed more than ever before. An integrated mental health service is one model of community-based care that is complex and requires integration of physical and mental health approaches to care. People with serious mental illness often lack attention to physical health needs, leading to chronic illness such as in diabetes, hypertension, and cardiovascular disease.[21] New antipsychotic medications have increased the incidence of these metabolic disorders. PMH RNs are optimal providers, given an education in integrated models of primary physical and mental health care delivery. PMH RNs are also successful negotiators within the fragmented health care system with multiple specialty providers, pharmacies, programs, and insurances.[17] Hoge and colleagues[4(p.22)] wrote, "It is difficult to overstate the magnitude of the workforce crisis in behavioral health."

Preparing a GPN Workforce

GPN evolved in the 1970s as a subspecialty of psychiatric nursing (an illness-oriented specialty) blended with gerontological nursing (focused more broadly on health and illness in older adults). Sixteen percent of psychiatric nurses have this subspecialty preparation in geriatrics and gerontology.[22] Advanced practice GPNs possess the knowledge to treat mental illness and to promote health and resiliency in diverse populations of elders living in a variety of care settings. The education of an advanced practice nurse in GPN begins with a 4-year baccalaureate degree in nursing and state licensure as an RN. Nurses then engage in a program of graduate studies that cover biobehavioral and pharmacologic sciences; recognition and diagnosis of common mental disorders; cognitive, behavioral, and interpersonal treatments; research; and other interests such as communication theory and practice, consultation, conflict resolution, and exposure to the ethical and legal issues unique to the treatment needs of older adults.[22] Meeting the complex physical and mental health care needs of elders in the decades ahead poses an enormous national and societal challenge, one in which GPN has an essential role to play.

Not all nurses will specialize as a GPN, but most of them will work with elders with mental health disorders. All nurses must therefore have a basic level of competency in GPN. The Geropsychiatric Nursing Collaborative (GPNC) was formed in 2006 to address this workforce shortage of GPN. A 2-pronged strategy was identified to address this need: GPN core competency enhancements and teaching resources for all nursing programs producing graduates who will work with older adults. GPNC has developed GPN core competency enhancements in partnership with key gerontological nursing organizations. The competency enhancements are designed to fit each type and level of nursing practice. The enhancements have been distributed to all nursing programs with graduates who care for older adults, nursing education journals, newsletters, and relevant national meetings. In addition, the identification and dissemination of GPN teaching resources promotes the inclusion of core GPN competencies at all levels of education. The GPNC Web site at www.aannet.org/GPNCgeropsych has many resources posted for education of nurses working with GPN populations.

Solutions to the Aging PMH RN Workforce

Never before have PMH RN employers been faced with the challenges of managing a nursing workforce in which most PMH RNs are older than 56 years (in 2009 data). Policies and practices most important to older PMH RN's decision to remain at work in organizations and the extent to which organizations engage in practices supportive of older nurses become much more important. Workplace changes may be necessary for a profession traditionally dominated by younger nurses. Hatcher and colleagues'[23] White Paper entitled Wisdom at Work: The Importance of the Older and Experienced Nurse in the Workplace gives a thorough review of the literature on older nurse retention (supplemented by surveys and interviews) undertaken by the Robert Wood Johnson Foundation. A baseline of best practices for retaining older nurses is provided, and future research to explore and develop fresh approaches is encouraged. The White Paper and compendium acknowledges successes to date and provides a challenge to health care organizations to make adjustments for the future.

Nursing literature suggests emerging commonalities in findings regarding older nurses' preferred work setting and intent to stay at work. A statewide survey in a small rural state found the oldest cohort (older than 61 years) of a sample of 4418 RNs to be the most stable and unlikely to leave their positions.[24] Older nurses were more likely to work part time and in settings of lesser acuity than the hospital. Creating career paths and the ability to delay retirement for a significant number of nurses may help facilitate a transition to a different work setting and thus help ease the shortage in the next decade. Evidence suggests that hospitals having the American Association of

Colleges of Nursing Magnet status recognition when compared with nonmagnet hospitals provided more support for their aging workforce. Hader and colleagues[25] found increased efforts to reduce physical strain, improve schedule flexibility, promote preventative care, establish succession planning, and offer educational/training opportunities. Nurse leaders were encouraged to design more innovative solutions for retaining older nurses while paying attention to keeping the workforce in generational balance. Val Palumbo and colleagues[26] used a survey to explore RNs' perceptions of their intentions to stay in their current position with their current employer. RNs (N = 583) planned to stay in the workforce slightly longer than they planned working as a nurse. The majority (58%) planned to continue working as a nurse after retirement. The top 3 human resource practices reported as important to their decision to remain in their present organizations were recognition and respect, having a voice, and receiving ongoing feedback regarding one's performance. These top 3 practices ranked above compensation and flexible work options. Notably, all 3 of these practices are within the management's control, resulting in the ability to retain older nurses. Smart organizations can position themselves as the choice employer by showing respect for the most experienced nurses' unique contributions.

SUMMARY

Although millions of Americans will thrive as they grow ever older, a dramatic increase in the number of people who survive to advanced old age means that there will be a dramatic increase in the number of elders who will experience chronic mental disorders. Health problems will include both physical and mental disorders and often situations where they co-occur. As survival to advanced old age occurs, so will devastating conditions such as Alzheimer disease. Meeting the complex needs for care for elders with mental disorders in the decades ahead will pose enormous national and societal challenges, especially to provide access to high-quality scientifically based GPNs. More resources and mental health services will be needed to meet the needs for access to care of the aging baby boom generation. Policy makers must anticipate not only the needs of the older population but also the removal of barriers to meeting these needs, such as the shortage of qualified health care providers.[22]

REFERENCES

1. Centers for Disease Control and Prevention. Public health and aging: trends in aging: United States and worldwide. 2003. Available at: http://www.cdc.gov/mmwr/preview/mmwrhtml/mm5206a2.htm. Accessed September 12, 2007.
2. Alzheimer's Association. 2009 Alzheimer's disease facts and figures: Alzheimer's & dementia. 2009. Available at: http://www.alz.org/national/documents/report_alzfactsfigures2009.pdf. Accessed March 6, 2009.
3. Clarke J. Adverse factors and the mental health of older people: implications for social policy and professional practice. J Psychiatr Ment Health Nurs 2005;12:290–6.
4. Hoge MA, Morris JA, Daniels AS, et al. An action plan for behavioral health workforce development. Cincinnati (OH): The Annapolis Coalition on the Behavioral Health Workforce; 2007. Available at: http://www.samhsa.rog/workforce/Annapolis/workforceactionplan.pdf. Accessed March 6, 2009.
5. Kelley SD. Prevalent mental health disorders in the aging population: issues of co morbidity and functional disability and substance abuse. The Journal of Rehabilitation 2003;69:19–25.

6. O'Sullivan CK, Krauss JB. True mental health parity: a long-overdue public health policy. Am J Nurs 2007;107:77–9.
7. Shern D. Parity pays dividends: increased costs in behavioral-health benefits offset by other savings. Mod Healthc 2009;39:24.
8. Husted E, Sharfstein SS, Muszionski S, et al. Reductions in coverage for mental and nervous illness in the Federal Employees Health Benefits Program 1980–1984. Am J Psychiatry 1985;142:181–6.
9. Barry CL. The political evolution of mental health parity. Harv Rev Psychiatry 2006;14:185–94.
10. Busch SH, Barry CL. New evidence on the effects of state mental health mandates. Inquiry 2008;45:308–22.
11. Dixon K. Implementing mental health parity: the challenge for health plans. Health Aff (Milwood) 2009;28(3):663–5.
12. Goldman HH. Behavioral health insurance parity for federal employees. N Engl J Med 2006;354(13):1378–86.
13. Barry CL, Ridgely MS. Mental health and substance abuse insurance parity for federal employees: how did heath plans respond? J Policy Anal Manage 2008; 27(1):155–70.
14. Trivedi AN, Swaminathan S, Mor V. Insurance parity and the use of outpatient mental health care following a psychiatric hospitalization. JAMA 2008;300(24): 2879–85.
15. Institute of Medicine of the National Academies. Retooling for an aging America: building the health care workforce. Washington, DC: The National Academies Press; 2008.
16. Buerhaus P. Peter Buerhaus talks about the nursing shortage. Creat Nurs 2008; 14:38–9.
17. Hanrahan MP. Analysis of the psychiatric mental health nurse workforce in the United States. J Psychosoc Nurs Ment Health Serv 2009;47(5):34–42.
18. Miller SD, Bausch S, Johnson B, et al. The registered nurse population: findings from the March 2004 national sample survey of registered nurses. Available at: http://bhpr.hrsa.gov/healthworkforce/msurvey04/. Accessed March 6, 2009.
19. National Association of Psychiatric Health Systems. New NAPHS annual survey tracks behavioral treatment trends. Available at. http://www.naphs.org/WhatsNew/documents/Annualsurvey2007.pdf. Accessed March 6, 2009.
20. Delaney KR, Johnson ME. Inpatient psychiatric nursing: why safety must be the key deliverable. Arch Psychiatr Nurs 2008;22:386–8.
21. Roberts KT, Robinson KM, Stewart C, et al. Integrated mental health practice in a nurse-managed health center. The American Journal for Nurse Practitioners 2008;12(10):33–47.
22. Kolanowski A, Piven ML. Geropsychiatric Nursing: The State of the Science. J Am Psychiatr Nurses Assoc 2006;12:75–99.
23. Hatcher BJ, Bleich MR, Connolly C, et al. Wisdom at work: the importance of the older and experienced nurse in the workplace. 2006. Available at: http://www.rwjf.org/files/publications/other/wisdomatwork.pdf. Accessed March 6, 2009.
24. McIntosh B, Rambur B, Palumbo MV, et al. The older nurse: clues for retention. Nurs Health Pol Rev 2003;2(2):1–18.
25. Hader R, Savwer C, Steltzer T. No time to lose. Nurs Manag 2006;37(7):23–6, 28–9, 48.
26. Val Palumbo M, McIntosh B, Rambur B, et al. Retaining an aging nurses workforce: perceptions of human resource practices. Nurs Econ 2009;27(4): 221–7, 232.

Assessing and Maintaining Mental Health in Elderly Individuals

Celeste Shawler, PhD, PMHCNS-BC

KEYWORDS

• Elderly individuals • Mental health • Assessment

Mental health and mental illness issues are as common later in life as they are at other ages. However, elderly adults are less likely to receive treatment for mental health issues and mental illness difficulties.[1] Depression and anxiety in older adults are frequently misinterpreted as a normal part of aging,[2] and assessment and treatment are not provided for older adults. The prevalence of delirium in hospitalized older adults ranges from 4% to 53.3%.[3] The syndrome of dementia includes many disorders such as Alzheimer disease, vascular dementia, Lewy body disease, and dementia resulting from head trauma.[4] An estimated 5.1 million people aged 65 years and older have Alzheimer disease.[5] Psychosis in the older adult may be caused from a diagnosis of schizophrenia, major depression, delirium, or substance abuse.[6] Psychosocial issues including abuse and neglect as well as substance abuse are a major concern for older adults. This article provides an overview of the mental health issues facing older adults. The mental health characteristics and the predominant mental illnesses in older adults are presented. Prevention, health promotion, assessment of mental health status, interventions, and resources for general nurses are discussed.

OVERVIEW OF MENTAL ILLNESSES AND MENTAL HEALTH ISSUES IN OLDER ADULTS

In the United States, about 3% of older adults experienced serious psychological stress in the past 30 days, and nearly 4% report serious psychological distress. Women are more likely to report symptoms of serious psychological distress.[7] The first United States Surgeon General Report on the global burden of disease[8] emphasizes that mental health and mental illness are critical concerns of individuals at all ages. Despite increased knowledge about the neuroscience of mental health, and improved treatments, key disparities persist for certain races and cultures, various ages, and between the genders. This report is a call to action for health providers

School of Nursing, University of Louisville, 555 South Floyd Street, Louisville, KY 40292, USA
E-mail address: c0shaw01@louisville.edu

Nurs Clin N Am 45 (2010) 635–650
doi:10.1016/j.cnur.2010.06.010
0029-6465/10/$ – see front matter © 2010 Elsevier Inc. All rights reserved.

nursing.theclinics.com

and all Americans to educate ourselves and others about mental health and mental illness and to eradicate the stigma and misunderstanding about mental illness. Nurses and all health care providers must increase their awareness and knowledge about mental health promotion and the specific illnesses and psychosocial issues facing older adults.

HEALTH AND MENTAL HEALTH PROMOTION IN OLDER ADULTS

Overall health promotion is important to the healthy functioning of the older adult. Specifically, health promotion involves immunizations, screenings, and counseling for health promotion behaviors.[9] The goal of health promotion is to maximize function and well-being in older adults.[10] Interventions that optimize mental health are crucial to maximize overall well-being and quality of life in the older adult. According to the United States Surgeon General's Report on Mental Illness,[8] there are many ways to prevent or reduce the risk of developing or exacerbating mental disorders. Primary prevention involves prevention of depression and suicide, excess disability, and unnecessary institutionalization. Most efforts are focused on prevention of depression and suicide in the older adult. Other avenues to promote mental health involve activities to increase long-term and short-term memory and interventions to preserve cognitive function with age.[11,12] A strategic plan to promote mental health and minimize disability from mental disorders, such as promotion of cognitive and emotional health and elimination of barriers to health promotion for older adults, including health disparities, is described in *Health indicators for healthy people 2010: mental health and mental disorders*.[13] The guide to clinical preventive services[14] includes quality improvement of programs to address mental health conditions and substance abuse issues; screening for dementia, depression, and suicidal risk; and screening for illicit and over-the-counter drug abuse.

Nurses and other health care providers should be knowledgeable about basic and specific screening strategies to prevent or reduce illness and promote well-being and mental health in older adults.[14] First, screening for mental health conditions and substance abuse in older adults can identify the need for behavioral counseling to reduce alcohol, illicit drug, or polypharmacy abuse. Second, the Mini-Mental State Examination (MMSE) is used to screen for dementia. A modified and updated version of the MMSE has been developed.[15] The MMSE is a widely used short instrument to quickly assess for cognitive impairment and its severity. Monitoring changes over time is also possible using the MMSE.[16–18] Third, nurses and health care providers must screen for depression and suicide risk. Because depression is common and often undetected and undiagnosed, screening to assess and institute proper treatment is essential to the well-being of the older adult. Depression assessment is described in detail later.

MENTAL HEALTH ASSESSMENT

Health care providers must have knowledge to conduct a comprehensive mental health assessment in older adults. There are multiple tools for screening various aspects of functioning such as physical performance, psychological functioning, affective, social, and psychosocial abilities. Comprehensive assessment can be conducted using the Fulmer SPICES assessment tool, which aids the health care provider to assess sleep disorders, problems with eating or feeding, incontinence, confusion, evidence of falls, and skin breakdown.[19] The General Assessment Series[20] *Try This: Best Practices in Nursing Care to Older Adults* includes 27 tools to assess a variety of conditions and situations in older adults. Examples of the tools are given in

Table 1. The Mini-Cog and sleep is assessed using the Pittsburgh Sleep Quality Index.[21] Also included in this series are tools to assess pain in the older adult, fall risk, and nutrition. In addition to assessment of the older adult, tools are available for use by nurses and health care providers to assess caregivers for strain using the modified Caregiver Strain Index (CSI). A new specialty practice series is being developed and 2 assessment tools are completed that aid providers to assess neuropathic pain in older adults and preparation for informal caregivers. The Try This Series has a Dementia Series that includes 11 tools and strategies to assess older adults with dementia. This compilation of assessment tools provides nurses and other health care providers with tools that are easy to use and administer. Use of these tools increases the specificity by which nurses and health care providers can assess older adults. These assessments increase awareness of the needs of older adults with a variety of illness symptoms and conditions.

COMMON PSYCHIATRIC ILLNESSES IN OLDER ADULTS
Depression

Of nearly 35 million Americans more than 65 years of age, an estimated 2 million have a depressive illness such as major depression, dysthymic disorder (chronic low mood), or bipolar disorder.[22] Depression is prevalent among older people and is estimated to affect between 8% and 20% of older adults in the community and up to 37% in primary care.[8] Depression in the older adult is often disguised by symptoms of physical discomfort and is one of the most common conditions associated with suicide in the older adult. Even though "older adults compromise about 12% of the US population, people age 65 and older accounted for 16% of suicide deaths in 2004."[23(p1)] Projections for occurrence of depression in 2020 for older adults indicate that it will be second only to heart disease as measured by global burden of disease.[24] The study of depression in older adults makes it clear that depression is not a normal part of aging and should be treated. Untreated depression can delay recovery or worsen outcomes of other comorbid illnesses in older adults.

Assessment
For an initial assessment, it has been documented that 2 questions provide reliable data to quickly assess the mood of older adults. These 2 questions are: (1) During the past month have you often been bothered by feeling down, depressed, or hopeless? (2) During the past month have you been bothered by little interest or pleasure in doing things?[25] If the older adult has a positive response to these questions, further detailed assessment should be conducted. Next, the nurse or health care provider should use the Geriatric Depression Scale in the General Assessment Series in the *Try This* series[20] to identify older adults who are depressed. In view of the prevalence of depression in the older adult, several general principles are helpful to accurately assess the older adult. First, in older adults, somatic complaints and the high prevalence of medical illnesses must be considered. Second, nonspecific or multiple somatic complaints may be suggestive of depression. Third, many drugs used to treat medical illnesses may potentially cause depressive symptoms. Fourth, always consult with psychiatric experts when there is uncertainty about the depression symptoms.[26] Because of the complexity of depression, somatic complaints, and often bereavement, depression scales should not be the sole assessment strategy. For example, if only the depression scales are used, the somatic complaints, which often indicate depression in older adults, will be missed.

Depressive disorders in older adults are often subthreshold disorders that include symptoms of depression, but they are not severe enough, nor frequent enough, to

Table 1
Examples of assessment tools

Assessment Tool	Functions Assessed
Fulmer SPICES	Sleep disorders, problems with eating or feeding, incontinence, confusion, evidence of falls, and skin breakdown
Katz Index of Independence in Activities of Daily Living (ADL)	Assess functional status of client's ability to perform activities of daily living of bathing, dressing, toileting, transferring, continence, and feeding
Geriatric Depression Scale (GDS)	30-item questionnaire in which older adults answer yes or no to how they have felt in the past week. Tool has 92% sensitivity and 89% specificity for diagnosing depression in older adults
Confusion Assessment Method (CAM)	CAM intended to provide standardization for clinicians to quickly and accurately identify delirium in clinical and research settings
Mini-Cog	Three-item recall and clock drawing to assess executive functioning
Pittsburgh Sleep Quality Index	Effective instrument used to measure quality and patterns of sleep in older adults. It differentiates poor from good sleep, helps identify sleep disturbances, use of sleeping medication, and daytime dysfunction in the last month
Modified Caregiver Strain Index (CSI)	A tool to quickly screen family caregivers to measure strain related to care provision. There are employment, financial, social, and time domains
Dementia series	Includes 11 tools specifically for assessing older adults with dementia. Examples include avoiding restraints with patients with dementia, assessing pain in persons with dementia, and recognition of dementia in hospitalized patients
CAM for intensive care units (CAM-ICU)	An adaptation of the CAM, the most widely used instrument for diagnosing delirium by nonpsychiatric clinicians. It is the only delirium assessment tool with yes/no questions for nonspeaking, mechanically ventilated patients in intensive care units (ICU)
Try This Executive Function	Tool for assessing executive function, and diagnosing previously undetected dementia in some older adults
Elder Mistreatment Assessment	41-item assessment instrument consisting of 7 sections that review signs, symptoms, and subjective complaints of elder abuse, neglect, exploitation, and abandonment

Printed with permission of The Hartford Institute for Geriatric Nursing, New York University, College of Nursing. Available on the internet at www.ConsultGeriRN. org/resources.

be diagnosed as depression.[27] Sadness, bereavement, fatigue, lack of appetite, and interference with sleep caused by physical illnesses may contribute to feelings of sadness and subthreshold depression. Being preoccupied with death may accompany a serious or terminal physical illness. Thus, when assessing depression in the older adult, the complexity of the clinical situation must be considered.

Because older adults with depression have a high suicide attempt and success rate, assessment of suicide ideation is essential in those who exhibit signs of depression. Assess suicide ideation by asking the older adult straightforward simple questions such as: Have you felt so sad, down, or depressed that you would hurt yourself?; Have you thought that you'd like to end it all? If the older adult responds positively to these questions, assessment of the means and plan to carry out the suicidal ideation is essential. Thus, the next questions would be: Do you have a plan?" and If so, what is it?" Based on responses, treatment should be initiated. Specific intervention strategies are discussed in the next section.

Nursing diagnoses

Potential nursing diagnoses for older adults with depression or depressive symptoms may include risk for self-directed violence, risk for self harm, disturbed thought processes, ineffective coping, interrupted family processes, hopelessness, powerlessness, situational low self-esteem, self-care deficit (hygiene/grooming/feeding/toileting/and so forth), and imbalanced nutrition.[28]

Interventions

Depression and misery in older adults are often considered to be a natural part of the aging process.[8] This viewpoint contributes to lack of diagnoses and vast undertreatment of depression in older adults. To change this viewpoint and practice, the goal for treatment of depression in older adults is to reduce and eliminate the symptoms, increase the quality of life, and improve functional status.[9,29,30] Psychosocial therapies, such as cognitive behavioral, interpersonal, and psychodynamic psychotherapies, can be effective with older adults. Individual, family, and group therapy can be provided by mental health professionals.[1,31–34] Additional treatment typically involves the use of pharmacotherapies in conjunction with psychotherapy. Antidepressants are generally an effective treatment of depression in older adults; however, there are special considerations for proper treatment. Specific guidelines for pharmacotherapy to treat depression in older adults should be followed.[35–37]

Delirium

Delirium is a common cause of acute confusion and morbidity and mortality.[38] Delirium is characterized by an acute cognitive impairment that develops in a few hours or days.[39]

The characteristics are disturbances in consciousness and cognition that cannot be explained by a known or developing dementia.[39] It is estimated that delirium complicates the hospitalized stays of more than 2.3 million older adults.[40] Prevalence rates of delirium in hospitalized older adults can be as high as 53%.[3]

Assessment

Assessment tools for delirium are provided by the Hartford Institute for Geriatric Nursing.[20] The Confusion Assessment Method (CAM) can be used to detect delirium.[41] This 11-item scale identifies the older adult who has an acute onset or fluctuating course of cognitive functioning, is inattentive, has disorganized thinking, or has an altered level of consciousness. There are multiple risk factors for delirium including advanced age, dementia, medical illness, multiple medications, alcohol abuse, depression, pain, sensory impairment, and increased blood urea nitrogen/creatinine ratio.[42]

Additional assessment tools are the CAM for intensive care units (CAM-ICU) and the baselines assessment Try This Executive Function. The CAM-ICU is an instrument that was intended for use by nonpsychiatrically trained clinicians to quickly identify delirium in the older adult in an ICU. The CAM-ICU is the only delirium assessment tool constructed with yes/no questions for use with nonspeaking, mechanically ventilated patients in ICUs. Sendelbach and Guthrie,[43] from the University of Iowa Gerontological Nursing Interventions Research Center, Research Translation and Dissemination Core, developed an evidence-based practice guideline for acute confusion. This guideline names assessment principles, assessment tools, preventive interventions, intervention principles, and multicomponent interventions for prevention of delirium. In addition, pharmaceutical interventions for treatment of delirium are recommended, such as prophylactic use of haloperidol to reduce the severity and duration of delirium and atypical antipsychotic medications to reduce the severity of delirium. Of utmost importance is the treatment of the cause of the delirium, such as infection, myocardial infarction, or other medical conditions such as hypoglycemia, hypercalcemia, hyponatremia, hypokalemia, and dehydration.[42] Among patients who are hospitalized, fractures, infections, malnutrition, 3 or more medications, neuroleptics and narcotics, male sex, age greater than 80 years, and bladder catheters can also contribute to the development of delirium.[26] In addition, delirium can be caused by fecal impaction or urinary retention.[44]

Nursing diagnoses
Delirium is characterized as an acute onset mental confusion. An example of a potential nursing diagnoses for older adults with delirium is an "acute confusion related to delirium of known (or unknown) etiology, as indicated by disorganized thinking, perceptual disturbances, impaired memory, difficulty focusing, inattention, and agitation."[45(p334)] Another nursing diagnosis could be impaired verbal communication.

Interventions
Accurate diagnosis is important so that appropriate interventions can be instituted. When the underlying conditions are identified and treated, the delirium generally reverses. However, while the older adult is being assessed and a differential diagnosis is being determined, there may be severe behaviors of agitation. Neuroleptic medication such as haloperidol can be used to treat these behaviors.[44] The safety and effectiveness of newer neuroleptic medications, such as risperidone, olanzapine, and quetiapine, are being investigated for effectiveness in treating agitation in delirium.[35,46] When using these medications, nurses need to carefully assess the older adult for signs of extrapyramidal side effects of the medications. Extrapyramidal side effects may consists of psuedoparkinsonism (masklike face, stiff and stooped posture), shuffling gait, and tremor. Other extrapyramidal side effects are acute dystonic reactions that involve acute contractions of tongue, face, neck, and back. Another symptom is akathisia, which is a motor-driven restlessness (for example, constant movement of limbs). Tardive dyskinesia can involve facial and lip movements, rapid movements of limbs, and jerking and twisting of the neck and shoulder. Immediate intervention is necessary for extrapyramidal side effects, including notification of medical staff, administration of benztropine (Cogentin), or diphyenhydramine (Benadryl).[47] The goal of the treatment is for the patient to be calmer, alert, and without side effects of the medication.[48]

There are a few studies on the effectiveness of interventions and treatments of delirium.[27,49] Findings indicated that modifiable factors are cognitive impairment, sleep deprivation, immobility, vision impairment, hearing impairment, and dehydration. Nursing adherence to all interventions proved to be statistically significant in a study by Inouye and colleagues.[49] Flaherty is studying the effects of a 24-hour delirium room among hospitalized elders. The delirium room includes 24-hour observation in a setting free of physical and chemical restraints. Although initial results do not present any evidence-based findings, the creative and exploratory nature of the research is significant for improving care of older adults with delirium.

Dementia

Dementia includes Alzheimer disease, dementia with Lewy bodies, and Parkinson dementia. Alzheimer disease is a major disorder for older adults and affects 8% to 15% of people more than 65 years of age.[5] Dementia is a clinical syndrome of cognitive deficits that involves both memory impairments and a disturbance in at least 1 other area of cognition (eg, aphasia, apraxia, agnosia) and disturbance in executive functioning.[39] In Alzheimer disease, there is a gradual, progressive loss of cognitive function including deficits in language, object and person recognition, and executive functioning.[8,50] Functional impairments in dementia include amnesia, aphasia, agnosia, and apraxia. Aphasia is language impairment and apraxia is inability to perform complex motor activities. Agnosia is the failure to recognize familiar objects or how to use them.[51] Alzheimer type dementia is typically classified into several stages: early, mid, and late. Early stage is characterized by gradual and subtle onset of symptoms. Midstage is characterized by worsening of recent and past memory. During late-stage Alzheimer disease the person becomes immobile, often bed or wheelchair confined, and muscles become rigid. Appetite is reduced and dysphagia is often present with increased risk of aspiration.[50,51]

Vascular dementia often presents with sudden onset and immediate changes in cognition.[51] Progression of vascular dementia is more stepwise than gradual and progressive as in Alzheimer disease. The individual with vascular dementia has the potential for multiple small strokes, with resultant changes in memory impairment.[51] Vascular dementia and delirium should be suspected with sudden onset of cognitive impairment.

Assessment

Several tools are helpful to screen for cognitive functioning, such as the Folstein MMSE[18] and the Mini-Cog[52] (see **Table 1**). In addition, the *Try This* dementia series has a subsection of specific tools to assess older adults with dementia. There are tools to guide nursing care that avoids use of restraints in persons with dementia as well as tools to assess pain. Other tools involve guides for therapeutic activity kits, assessment of wandering in the hospitalized older adult, and assessment of communication difficulties in the person with dementia.

In addition to cognitive impairment in individuals with dementia, neuropsychiatric symptoms are common. These symptoms can include agitation, aggression, hallucinations, repetitive vocalizations, wandering, and often depression.[53]

Nursing diagnoses

There are several possibilities of nursing diagnoses related to the older person with dementia. One diagnosis is risk for injury related to sensory dysfunction, cognitive or emotional difficulties, biochemical processes, and confusion.[28] Another diagnosis is "self-care deficit related to cognitive impairment, confusion, apraxia and severe memory impairment."[28(p403)] A key nursing diagnosis involves "impaired verbal communication related to decreased circulation in the brain, deterioration or damage to the neurologic centers in the brain, severe memory impairment, escalating anxiety."[28(p406)] Including family members in the nursing care is essential when an older adult is diagnosed with dementia. A nursing diagnosis that may be helpful is "caregiver role strain, related to duration of caregiving, caregiver isolation, and 24-hour care responsibility."[28(p410)]

Interventions

Many resources are available to guide interventions for older adults with dementia. Nursing care strategies from the Hartford Institute for Geriatric Nursing[54] provide comprehensive, evidence-based practice, and descriptive information. For example, clinical experts and scholars recommend that nurses monitor the side effects of medications used in older adults to improve cognitive functioning. Techniques to enhance cognitive functioning and social engagement are essential. It is critically important to monitor and ensure that the older adult with dementia has adequate fluids, nutrition, comfort measures, and rest. Physical and pharmacologic restraints should be avoided if possible while enhancing mobility and functional capacity. Address behavioral issues and attend to environmental situations that trigger confusion or agitation. Provide reassurance, redirect, limit stimuli, respect space, and refer as needed to mental health care professionals. Always make sure the environment is therapeutic and safe and provides a balance of stimulation and relaxation. Safety measures include name tags, medic alert systems, and wander alarms. Nursing care should be consistent and predictable. Nurses should assist with individuals with dementia and advise their family members about advance-care planning and end-of-life care. Caregiver education and support are essential.

Anxiety

Anxiety in older adults often resembles physical illness and thus is often underrecognized and undertreated.[9,55] It is estimated that about 11.4% of adults more than 55 years old meet criteria for an anxiety disorder.[55] Anxiety disorders consist of phobic anxiety disorders, panic disorder, posttraumatic stress disorder (PTSD), and obsessive-compulsive disorder.[8,55,56] Worry and nervous tension are likely to be reported by older adults. It is estimated that PTSD will increase with the aging of Vietnam veterans and veterans with combat exposure.[8]

Assessment

Detection of anxiety in older adults is confounded by high medical comorbidity, polypharmacy, and difficulty distinguishing depression from anxiety.[55] Anxiety and depression in later life are difficult to assess and differentiate. Beekman and colleagues[57] found that older adults often met the criteria for anxiety and depression simultaneously. These researchers recommended that pure anxiety disorders in the older adult needed further study. Onset of generalized anxiety disorder (GAD) in older adults typically occurs in late life. However, those with early onset of GAD may have a more difficult course in later life.[58]

Comprehensive assessment of older adults should include clinical interviews and evaluations, self-report measurement scales, and descriptive evidence. Self-report measurement scales include the Beck Depression Inventory. The psychometric properties of this inventory were validated by Segal and colleagues,[59] who found that the Beck Depression Inventory had strong psychometric support as a screening measure for older adults. Because anxiety symptoms in older adults often present as physical illnesses, screening and differentiating from physical and drug related symptoms is essential. Comprehensive assessment of over-the-counter and prescription medication, along with caffeine intake, is essential.[9]

Nursing diagnoses

Examples of diagnoses that could be used for older adults with diagnosed anxiety disorders include the following: "Anxiety, related to persistent chronic worry about multiple daily events or situations, as indicated by muscle tension, difficulty controlling worries, interference with functioning, and sleep disturbances."[45(p302)] If a major symptom is sleep difficulties, appropriate nursing diagnoses might be "sleep deprivation, related to prolonged chronic anxiety state, as indicated by fatigue, reports of difficulty sleeping and nervousness."[45(p303)] Lack of control of anxiety could lead to powerlessness. Thus an appropriate nursing diagnosis would be "powerlessness related to difficulty controlling anxiety and worry, as indicated by continued feelings of worry, interference with functional level, and effect on sleeping."[45(p305)]

Interventions

Few older adults with mental health difficulties use mental health services[60]; therefore astute assessment and appropriate interventions in primary care are important with older adults. Referral to psychiatric specialists is essential for thorough assessment, diagnosis, and treatment. Pharmacologic interventions can be helpful. Frequently selective serotonin reuptake inhibitors and serotonin and norepinephrine reuptake inhibitors are used for older adults.[55] In addition, cognitive behavior therapy (CBT) can be helpful for older adults with GAD. In a randomized clinical trial of 134 older adults in primary care settings, older adults receiving CBT showed greater improvement in depressive symptoms and general mental health.[61] Other researchers explored interventions that might prevent symptoms of depression and anxiety in older adults. In a randomized clinical trial, interventions addressed subclinical symptoms of depression and anxiety of older adults. Older adults receiving the preventive CBT-based bibliotherapy and problem-solving treatment were more likely to show improvement than those in the control group.[62]

Psychosis

Psychosis is currently recognized as a compilation of symptoms that occur in several physical and mental states in older adults. Characteristics of psychosis include hallucinations (false sensory perceptions) and delusions (false beliefs).[39] Older adults who have had chronic psychosis typically have been diagnosed with schizophrenia, major depression, or bipolar disorder with psychosis.[6] Psychoses in the older adult may be a symptom of delirium, substance use or abuse, or polypharmacy or mood disorder with psychotic features.

Assessment

An interdisciplinary team approach should be used systematically for the assessment and should include the older adult, the family, and other health care providers involved in the care of the older adult. First, the clinician should determine whether the psychosis is primary (schizophrenia, bipolar disorders, psychotic depression) or secondary (delirium, psychotic symptoms associated with dementia, and caused by a medical condition or drug interaction).[36] Overall assessment should include appearance, mood and affect, sensorium, intellectual function, and thought processes. Assessment should include chief complaint, history of illness, past psychiatric history, past medical history, substance abuse history, current and past medications, current lifestyle, cultural background, residence, mental status, and sensorium.[12]

Nursing diagnoses

There are multiple nursing diagnoses that may be pertinent for the older adult with psychosis. Examples include disturbed sensory perception related to neurologic disturbances, as indicated by hallucinations; and distorted thinking and disturbed thought processes related to possible neurochemical dysregulation, as indicated by non–reality-based thinking, thought blocking, broadcasting, hallucinations, delusions, and speech disturbances.[38] In addition, always consider the risk for suicide in older adults. A nursing diagnosis pertinent to this situation could be risk for suicide related to behavioral, situational, psychological, or social factors.[63]

Interventions

Jung and Newton[64] identified 28 interventions after a systematic search and review of the Cochrane reviews for schizophrenia, psychosis, schizoaffective, and bipolar disorders. This review summarizes findings from multiple studies where the effectiveness of interventions for older adults was analyzed. Interventions included art and drama therapy, cognitive rehabilitation, multidisciplinary team approaches, hypnosis, life-skill programs, and different environmental living situations.

Antipsychotic pharmacologic treatment is typically the choice for older adults with psychosis. Linton and Lach[12] provide information about the routes, and possible side effects, of medications such as haloperidol, clozapine, olanzapine, risperidone, zipraisidone, and quetiapine. Nursing interventions must include assessment and treatment of extrapyramidal side effects such as parkinsonian syndrome, akathisia, and tardive dyskinesia. Broadway and Mintzer[65] reported that antipsychotic drugs did improve the psychotic symptoms in the elderly, but the side effects may outweigh the benefits. Marriott, Neil, and Weddingham[66] searched the Cochrane Schizophrenia Group's Register (May 2003) and collected data related to antipsychotic treatment of older adults with schizophrenia. Findings indicated few robust data to guide clinicians in the appropriate pharmacologic treatment. The principles that should guide pharmacotherapy include thorough assessment of the older adult, determination of the type of psychosis, and appropriate choice of medication and awareness of side effects.[6] Additional nursing interventions for psychosis include crisis intervention, especially if the older adult is a danger to self or others, and evidence-based individual and group interventions.[6]

Psychosocial

Psychosocial issues of older adults include abuse and neglect as well as substance abuse. Abuse can be in the form of physical, sexual, emotional or psychological, neglect, abandonment, self-neglect, and financial or material exploitation.[67,68] Physical abuse is characterized by evidence of physical force that typically results in injury to the body causing pain or impairment. Symptoms of physical abuse include unexplained bruises, burns, fractures, lacerations, or abrasions. Sexual abuse is suspected when an older individual is forced to engage in sexual acts, is raped, is touched without consent, and coerced into nudity and explicit photographing. Signs and symptoms of sexual abuse are difficulty walking, pain or itching in genital area, and bruises or bleeding in external genitalia, vaginal, or anal areas. Emotional and psychological abuse is characterized by infliction of pain or distress through verbal or nonverbal communication. Suspected behaviors that indicate emotional abuse in older adults include sleep disorders, speech disturbances, conduct disorder, hysteria, obsessions, or hypochrondria.[51,69,70]

Neglect can involve caregiver and self-neglect, and these have similar presentations. Manifestations of neglect in the older adult include malnourishment, poor hygiene, inadequate clothing, unsafe and/or unclean living conditions, oversedation, and being left unattended.[69,70] Abandonment involves "the desertion of an older person by an individual who has physical custody of the elder or by a person who has assumed responsibility for providing care to an elder."[51(p287)] Financial and material exploitation involves illegal or improper use of an elder's property, assets, and material belongings.[70] Examples of financial abuse include forcing an elder to write checks, forging signatures, stealing money or possessions, and improper and dishonest use of power-of-attorney privileges.

Diagnosis of substance abuse in the older adult includes assessment of increased tolerance of the effects of substance use, which results in increased consumption.[23] See *Substance Use by Older Adults: Estimates of Future Impact on the Treatment System* from the Substance Abuse and Mental Health Services Administration (SAMHSA) Office of Applied Studies[71] for more information about the significance of substance abuse issues for older adults.

Assessment

Physical assessment of older adults for possible abuse and neglect should include general appearance, assessment of the musculoskeletal, neurologic, genital/rectal systems, and psychological response to abuse. The head, neck, skin, breasts, and genital/rectal areas should be inspected. Physical signs of abuse should be photographed.[70,72] In addition, a variety of assessment and screening tools are available to nurses, such as the Hartford *Try This* series: *Elder Mistreatment Assessment*.[73] A tool for screening women and elderly adults for family and intimate partner violence[74] is available online. Wolfe[75] has excellent assessment questions and explanations for clinicians collecting information from older adults when there is suspected abuse. Fulmer and colleagues[76] provide a summary of assessment instruments for elder abuse screening.

Nursing diagnoses

A possible nursing diagnosis is risk for injury related to violence or neglect, as indicated by recurrent emergency department visits, insomnia, bruises of various stages of healing, broken bones, scars, burns, malnutrition, and wounds. A diagnosis related to psychological abuse could be powerlessness and fear related to family, and caregiver abuse as indicated by feelings of shame and worthlessness, depression, helplessness, and low self-esteem. Another diagnosis could be related to rape and trauma such as rape-trauma syndrome related to sexual abuse as indicated by vaginal/anal bleeding, sores, bruises, and peritoneal pain.[28]

Interventions

Nurses have a legal responsibility to report suspected elder abuse.[47] An interdisciplinary team approach should be used to plan comprehensive interventions for an older person who has been abused or neglected. After diagnosis, referral to Adult Protective Services is needed.[47,69] The physical needs, such as nutrition and care of physical injuries, should be met. Psychological needs may require referral to appropriate mental health counseling centers. Nurses need to collaborate with the older adult to develop safety plans and a written list of emergency numbers and referrals; education about abuse is also essential. In addition, if abuse and neglect are suspected, address these issues with caregivers, and simultaneously evaluate caregivers for distress and drug and/or alcohol problems. Caregivers should be referred to drug/alcohol rehabilitation programs as appropriate.[70]

RESEARCH AND EVIDENCE-BASED RESOURCES

Many resources are readily available to nurse clinicians as they care for older adults and work to achieve maximum mental health status. Examples of resources to guide practice are outlined in this section.

Bartels and colleagues[77] conducted a systematic review and meta-analysis of evidence-based practices in geriatric mental health care. The investigators summarized the evidence-based practices for recognizing and treating depression, behavioral symptoms of dementia, schizophrenia, and anxiety disorders in older adults.

Jung and Newton[64] summarized the Cochrane reviews of non–medication-based psychotherapeutic and other interventions for schizophrenia, psychosis, and bipolar disorder in adults. Although not specific for older adults, the findings from this review provide a helpful resource. Rabins and colleagues[1] evaluated the effectiveness of a nurse-based outreach program for treating psychiatric illnesses in the elderly. A program entitled Psychogeriatric Assessment and Treatment in City Housing (PATCH) was studied in a randomized trial with 371 participants living in 6 public housing sites for elderly persons. The PATCH model and treatment consisted of monitoring vital signs and medication side effects, counseling, patient education, liaison with the on-site social service worker, and supervision of patients' compliance with medication. Results indicated that older persons treated with the intervention had lower ratings on the Montgomery-Asberg Depression Rating Scale, as well as lower scores on the Brief Psychiatric Rating Scale than those in the nontreatment comparison groups.

The Hartford Institute for Geriatric Nursing (ConsultGeriRN.org) has many evidence-based geriatric topics with thorough directions on assessment, risk factors, and treatment of many health issues for older adults. Assessment tools, instructional videos for the assessment tools, and suggestions for treatment are included at http://consultgerirn.org/. Another resource of interest is the Evidence-Based Protocol for Atypical Presentation.[78] Because illness in older adults is complicated by physical and mental changes, nurses must recognize atypical presentations of illness. For example, the investigators state that a diminished appetite and decrease in function in an older adult may be the first sign of illness. This resource is valuable to nurses and health care providers of older adults in the community and primary care, as well as older adults hospitalized for acute illnesses or exacerbations of chronic illnesses.

In conclusion, older adults deserve astute, accurate, and excellent mental health care. In the last years of their lives, older adults should have access to clinicians who are knowledgeable and use evidence-based practice. Future demographic trends indicate that many older adults will be living with multiple mental health needs along with physical needs. It is of supreme importance that health professionals provide caring, knowledgeable, and comprehensive care to older adults to ensure successful aging.

REFERENCES

1. Rabins PV, Black BX, Roca R, et al. Effectiveness of a nurse-based outreach program for identifying and treating psychiatric illness in the elderly. JAMA 2000;283(21):2803–9.
2. Henderson J. Aging and public health. In: Dharmarajan T, Norman R, editors. Clinical geriatrics. New York: Parthenon Publishing; 2003. p. 1–8.
3. Bruce A, Ritchie CW, Blizard R, et al. The incidence of delirium associated with orthopedic surgery: a meta-analytic review. Int Psychogeriatr 2007;19(2): 197–214.

4. Raskind MA, Bonner LT, Peskind ER. Cognitive disorders. In: Blazer DG, Steffens DC, Busse EW, editors, Textbook of geriatric psychiatry, 3. Washington, DC: American Psychiatric Publishing; 2004. p. 207–29.

5. Alzheimer's Disease Facts and Figures. Available at: http://www.alz.org/documents_custom/report_alzfactsfigures2010.pdf. Accessed May 8, 2010.

6. Mentes C, Bail JK. Psychosis in older adults. In: Melillo KD, Houde SC, editors. Geropsychiatric and mental health nursing. Sudbury (MA): Jones and Bartlett; 2005. p. 173–8.

7. Schoenborn CA, Heyman KM. Health characteristics of adults aged 55 years and over: United States, 2004–2007. National Health Statistics Reports; no.16. Hyattsville (MD): National Center for Health Statistics; 2009.

8. US Department of Health and Human Services. Mental health: a report of the surgeon general. Rockville (MD): US Department of Health and Human Services, Substance Abuse and Mental Health Services Administration, Center for Mental Health Services, National Institutes of Health, National Institute of Mental Health; 1999.

9. Molony SL, Waszynski CM, Lyder CH. Gerontological nursing: an advanced practice approach. Stamford (CT): Appleton & Lange; 1999.

10. Albert ST. Public health and aging: an introduction to maximizing function and well-being. New York: Springer; 2004.

11. Aberg AC, Sidenvall B, Hepworth M, et al. On loss of activity and independence, adaptation improves life satisfaction in old age – a qualitative study of patients' perceptions. Qual Life Res 2005;14:1111–25.

12. Linton AD, Lach HW. Gerontological nursing: concepts and practice. 3rd edition. St Louis (MO): Saunders Elsevier; 2007.

13. Healthy People. 2010. Available at: http://www.healthypeople.gov/lhi/lhiwhat.htm. Accessed April 17, 2010.

14. US Department of Health and Human Services. Guide to clinical preventive services. Available at: http://www.ahrq.gov/clinic/cps3dix.htm#mental. Accessed May 5, 2010.

15. Teng EL, Chui HC. The Modified Mini Mental State (3MS) examination. J Clin Psychiatry 1987;48:314–8.

16. Borson S, Scanlan J, Brush M, et al. The Mini-Cog: a cognitive 'vital signs' measure for dementia screening in multi-lingual elderly. Int J Geriatr Psychiatry 2000;15(11):1021–7.

17. Crum RM, Anthony JC, Bassett SS, et al. Population-based norms for the Mini-Mental State Examination by age and educational level. JAMA 1993;269(18):2386–91.

18. Folstein MF, Folstein SE, McHugh PR. Mini-Mental State: a practical method for grading the cognitive state of patients for the clinician. J Psychiatr Res 1975; 12:89–198.

19. Wallace M, Fulmer T. Fulmer SPICES: an overall assessment tool for older adults. Try This series: best practices in nursing care to older adults from the Hartford Institute for Geriatric Nursing. New York: New York University, College of Nursing; 2007. Available at: http://consultgerirn.org/uploads/File/trythis/issue01.pdf. Accessed December 18, 2009.

20. Hartford Institute for Geriatric Nursing. ConsultGeriRN.org assessment tools - Try This:® and How to Try This resources. Available at: http://consultgerirn.org/resources. Accessed May 7, 2010.

21. Buysse DJ, Reynolds CF, Monk TH, et al. The Pittsburgh Sleep Quality Index (PSQI): a new instrument for psychiatric research and practice. Psychiatry Res 1989;28:193–213.

22. Anxiety disorders research at the National institute of mental health. 2009. Available at: http://www.stress-anxiety-depression.org/anxiety/anxiety-disorders-research-nimh.html. Accessed April 10, 2010.

23. National Institute of Mental Health. Older adults: depression and suicide facts (fact sheet). (NIH Publication No. 4593). Available at: http://www.nimh.nih.gov/health/publications/older-adults-depression-and-suicide-facts-fact-sheet/index.shtml. Accessed May 7, 2010.

24. Chapman DP, Perry GS. Depression as a major component of public health for older adults. Preventing chronic disease: public health research, practice, and policy. 2008 [cited 2010 May 7]; 5(1): [about 2p]. Available at: www.cdc.gov/pcd/issues/2008/jan/07_0150.htm. Accessed February 7, 2010.

25. Arroll B, Khin N, Kerse N. Screening for depression in primary care with two verbally asked questions: cross sectional study. Br Med J 2003;327:1144–6.

26. Kane RL, Ouslander JG, Abrass IB. Essentials of clinical geriatrics. 5th edition. New York: McGraw-Hill; 2004.

27. Flaherty E, Fulmer T, Mezey M, editors. Geriatric nursing review syllabus: a core curriculum in advanced practice geriatric nursing. New York: American Geriatrics Society; 2003.

28. Varcarolis EM. Manual of psychiatric nursing care plans: diagnoses, clinical tools, and psychopharmacology. St Louis (MO): Saunders Elsevier; 2006.

29. Gallo JJ, Bogner HR, Fulmer T, et al. Handbook of geriatric assessment. 4th edition. Sudbury (MA): Jones and Barlett; 2006.

30. Lach HW. Health promotion and health education for older adults. In: Linton AD, Lach HW, editors. Gerontological nursing: concepts and practice. 3rd edition. St Louis (MO): Saunders Elsevier; 2007. p. 785–808.

31. Ell K. Depression care for elderly: reducing barriers to evidence based practice. Home Health Care Serv Q 2006;25:115–48.

32. Kurlowicz LH. Nursing standard of practice protocol: depression. Hartford Institute for Geriatric Nursing. 2008. Available at: http://consultgerirn.org/topics/depression/want_to_know_more. Accessed April 5, 2010.

33. Kurlowicz LH, Harvath TA. Depression. In: Capezuti E, Zwicker D, Mezey M, et al, editors. Evidence-based geriatric nursing protocols for best practice. 3rd edition. New York: Springer; 2008. p. 57–82.

34. Whelan-Gales MA, Griffin MT, Maloni J, et al. Spiritual well-being, spiritual practices, and depressive symptoms among elderly patients hospitalized with acute heart failure. Geriatr Nurs 2009;30:312–7.

35. Kurlowicz LH. Delirium and depression. In: Cotter VT, Strumpf NE, editors. Advanced practice nursing with older adults: clinical guidelines. New York: McGraw-Hill; 2002.

36. Melillo KD, Houde SC, editors. Geropsychiatric and mental health nursing. Sudbury (MA): Jones and Bartlett; 2005.

37. Unutzer J, Katon W, Callahan CM, et al. Depression treatment in a sample of 1,801 depressed older adults in primary care. J Am Geriatr Soc 2010;51:505–14.

38. Rizzo JA, Bogardus ST, Leo-Summers L, et al. A multicomponent targeted intervention to prevent delirium in hospitalized older patients: what is the economic value? Med Care 2001;39:740–52.

39. American Psychiatric Association. Diagnostic and statistical manual of mental disorders. 4th edition. Washington, DC: American Psychiatric Association; 2000.

40. Inouye SK, Bogardus ST, Charpentier PA, et al. A multicomponent intervention to prevent delirium in hospitalized older patients. N Engl J Med 1999;340:669–76.

41. Waszynski CM. The confusion assessment method (CAM). Try This series: best practices in nursing care to older adults from the Hartford Institute for Geriatric Nursing. New York: New York University, College of Nursing; 2007.

42. Tullmann DF, Mion LD, Fletcher K, et al. Nursing standard of practice protocol: delirium: prevention, early recognition, and treatment. Hartford Institute for Geriatric Nursing. 2008. Available at: http://consultgerirn.org/topics/delirium/want_to_know_more. Accessed January 22, 2010.

43. Sendelbach S, Guthrie PF. Evidence-based practice guideline: acute confusion/delirium. Iowa City (IA): University of Iowa Gerontological Nursing Interventions Research Center, Research Translation and Dissemination Core; 2009.

44. Millsap P. Neurological system. In: Linton AD, Lach HW, editors. Gerontological nursing: concepts and practice. 3rd edition. St Louis (MO): Saunders Elsevier; 2007. p. 406–38.

45. Foley M. Lippincott's handbook for psychiatric nursing and care planning. Philadelphia: Lippincott Williams & Wilkins; 2010.

46. Hwang J, Yang C, Lee T, et al. The efficacy and safety of olanzapine for the treatment of geriatric psychosis. J Clin Psychopharmacol 2003;23:113–8.

47. Inouye SK. Delirium. In: Cassel CK, editor. Geriatric medicine: an evidence-based approach. New York: Springer-Verlag; 2003. p. 1113–22.

48. Varcarolis EM, Carson VB, Shoemaker NC, editors. Foundations of psychiatric and mental health nursing: a clinical approach. 5th edition. St Louis (MO): Saunders Elsevier; 2006.

49. Inouye SK, Bogardus ST, Williams CS, et al. The role of adherence on the effectiveness of nonpharmacologic interventions. Arch Intern Med 2003;163:958–64.

50. Evans L. Complex care needs in older adults with common cognitive disorders. Section A: assessment and management of dementia. 2007. Available at: http://hartfordign.org/uploads/File/gnec_state_of_science_papers/gnec_dementia.pdf. Accessed December 14, 2009.

51. Stanley M, Blair KA, Beare PG. Gerontological nursing: promoting successful aging with older adults. 3rd edition. Philadelphia: FA Davis; 2005.

52. Borson S, Scanlan JM, Watanabe J, et al. Improving identification of cognitive impairment in primary care. Int J Geriatr Psychiatry 2005;21:349–55.

53. Lyketsos CG, Colenda CC, Beck C, et al. Position statement of the American Association for Geriatric Psychiatry regarding principles of care for patients with dementia resulting from Alzheimer disease. Am J Geriatr Psychiatry 2006; 14(7):561–73.

54. Hartford Institute for Geriatric Nursing: your portal to geriatric nursing resources. 2008. Available at: http://consultgerirn.org/resources. Accessed May 2, 2010.

55. Lauderdale S, Sheikh JI. Anxiety disorders in older adults. Clin Geriatr Med 2003; 19:21–741.

56. Busutill W. Presentation and management of post traumatic stress disorder and the elderly: a need for investigation. Int J Geriatr Psychiatry 2004;19:429–39.

57. Beekman AT, deBeurs E, vanBalkom AJ, et al. Anxiety and depression in later life: co-occurrence and communality of risk factors. Am J Psychiatry 2000;157:89–95.

58. LeRoux H, Gatz M, Wetherell JL. Age at onset of generalized anxiety disorder in older adults. Am J Geriatr Psychiatry 2005;13(1):23–30.

59. Segal D, Coolidge FL, Cahill BS, et al. Psychometric properties of the Beck Depression Inventory-II (BDI-II) among community dwelling older adults. Behav Modif 2008;32(1):3–20.

60. Klap R, Unroe KT, Unutzer J. Caring for mental illness in the United States: a focus on older adults. Am J Geriatr Psychiatry 2003;11(5):517–624.

61. Stanley M, Wilson NL, Novy DM, et al. Cognitive behavior therapy for generalized anxiety disorder among older adults in primary care: a randomized clinical trial. JAMA 2009;301(14):1460–7.
62. van't Veer-Tazelaar PJ, van Marwijk HW, van Oppen P, et al. Stepped-care prevention of anxiety and depression in late life. Arch Gen Psychiatry 2009; 66(3):207–304.
63. North American Nurses Diagnosis Association. Nursing diagnosis: definitions and classifications 2005–2006. Philadelphia: NANDA International; 2005.
64. Jung XT, Newton R. Cochrane reviews of non-medication-based psychotherapeutic and other interventions for schizophrenia, psychosis and bipolar disorder: a systematic literature review. Int J Ment Health Nurs 2009;18:239–49.
65. Broadway J, Mintzer J. The many faces of psychosis in the elderly. Curr Opin Psychiatry 2007;20(4):551–8.
66. Marriott R, Neil W, Waddingham S. Antipsychotic medication for elderly people with schizophrenia. Cochrane database Syst Rev 2006;1:CD005580.
67. Fulmer T, Guadagno L, Bolton MM. In: Melillo KD, Houde SC, editors. Geropsychiatric and mental health nursing. Sudbury (MA): Jones and Bartlett; 2005.
68. National Center on Elder Abuse. Administration on aging. 2008. Available at: http://www.ncea.aoa.gov/NCEAroot/Main_Site/FAQ/Basics/Types_Of_Abuse. aspx. Accessed May 15, 2010.
69. Cotter VT, Strumpf NE, editors. Advanced practice nursing with older adults: clinical guidelines. New York: McGraw-Hill; 2002.
70. Fulmer T, Greenberg S. Elder mistreatment and abuse: Hartford Institute for Geriatric Nursing. Available at: http://consultgerirn.org/topics/elder_mistreatment_and_abuse/want_to_know_more; 2008. Accessed May 24, 2010.
71. Substance Abuse and Mental Health Services Administration (SAMHSA): Office of Applied Studies. Substance use by older adults: estimates of future impact on the treatment system. Available at: http://www.oas.samhsa.gov/aging/toc. htm. Accessed May 26, 2010.
72. Wagner L, Greenberg S, Capezuti E. Elder abuse and neglect. In: Cotter VT, Strumpf NE, editors. Advanced practice nursing with older adults: clinical guidelines. New York: McGraw-Hill; 2002. p. 319–32.
73. Fulmer T. Elder mistreatment assessment: Try This series. Hartford Center for Geriatric Nursing. 2008. Available at: http://consultgerirn.org/resources. Accessed May 25, 2010.
74. Nelson H, Nygren P, McInerney Y, et al. Screening women and elderly adults for family and intimate partner violence: a review of the evidence for the U.S. preventive services task force. Ann Intern Med 2004;140(5):387–96 Agency for Healthcare Research and Quality, Rockville (MD). Available at: http://www.ahrq.gov/clinic/3rduspstf/famviolrev.htm. Accessed February 14, 2010.
75. Wolf R. Risk assessment instruments. Special research review section of the national Center on Elder Abuse. 2000. Available at: http://www.ncea.aoa.gov/Main_Site/Library/Statistics_Research/Research_Reviews/riskassessment.aspx. Accessed May 10, 2010.
76. Fulmer T, Guadagno L, Dyer CB, et al. Progress in elder abuse screening and assessment instruments. J Am Geriatr Soc 2004;52(2):297–304.
77. Bartels SJ, Dums AR, Oxman TE, et al. Evidence-based practices in geriatric mental health care. Journal of Lifelong Learning in Psychiatry 2004;11:268–81.
78. Flaherty E, Zwicker D. Atypical presentation. 2005. Available at: http://consultgerirn.org/topics/atypical_presentation/want_to_know_more. Accessed June 1, 2010.

Index

Nurs Clin N Am 45 (2010) 651–660
doi:10.1016/S0029-6465(10)00088-5
0029-6465/10/$ – see front matter © 2010 Elsevier Inc. All rights reserved.

nursing.theclinics.com

United States Postal Service

Statement of Ownership, Management, and Circulation
(All Periodicals Publications Except Requestor Publications)

1. Publication Title	2. Publication Number								3. Filing Date
Nursing Clinics of North America	5	9	9	8	-	9	6	0	0	9/15/10

4. Issue Frequency	5. Number of Issues Published Annually	6. Annual Subscription Price
Mar, Jun, Sep, Dec	4	$133.00

7. Complete Mailing Address of Known Office of Publication (*Not printer*) (*Street, city, county, state, and ZIP+4®*)

Elsevier Inc.
360 Park Avenue South
New York, NY 10010-1710

Contact Person
Stephen Bushing

Telephone (*Include area code*)
215-239-3688

8. Complete Mailing Address of Headquarters or General Business Office of Publisher (*Not printer*)

Elsevier Inc., 360 Park Avenue South, New York, NY 10010-1710

9. Full Names and Complete Mailing Addresses of Publisher, Editor, and Managing Editor (*Do not leave blank*)

Publisher (*Name and complete mailing address*)

Kim Murphy, Elsevier, Inc., 1600 John F. Kennedy Blvd. Suite 1800, Philadelphia, PA 19103-2899

Editor (*Name and complete mailing address*)

Katie Hartner, Elsevier, Inc., 1600 John F. Kennedy Blvd. Suite 1800, Philadelphia, PA 19103-2899

Managing Editor (*Name and complete mailing address*)

Catherine Bewick, Elsevier, Inc., 1600 John F. Kennedy Blvd. Suite 1800, Philadelphia, PA 19103-2899

10. Owner (*Do not leave blank. If the publication is owned by a corporation, give the name and address of the corporation immediately followed by the names and addresses of all stockholders owning or holding 1 percent or more of the total amount of stock. If not owned by a corporation, give the names and addresses of the individual owners. If owned by a partnership or other unincorporated firm, give its name and address as well as those of each individual owner. If the publication is published by a nonprofit organization, give its name and address.*)

Full Name	Complete Mailing Address
Wholly owned subsidiary of	4520 East-West Highway
Reed/Elsevier, US holdings	Bethesda, MD 20814

11. Known Bondholders, Mortgagees, and Other Security Holders Owning or Holding 1 Percent or More of Total Amount of Bonds, Mortgages, or Other Securities. If none, check box. ☐ None

Full Name	Complete Mailing Address
N/A	

12. Tax Status (*For completion by nonprofit organizations authorized to mail at nonprofit rates*) (*Check one*)
The purpose, function, and nonprofit status of this organization and the exempt status for federal income tax purposes:
☐ Has Not Changed During Preceding 12 Months
☐ Has Changed During Preceding 12 Months (*Publisher must submit explanation of change with this statement*)

PS Form 3526, September 2007 (Page 1 of 3 (Instructions Page 3)) PSN 7530-01-000-9931 PRIVACY NOTICE: See our Privacy policy in www.usps.com

13. Publication Title		14. Issue Date for Circulation Data Below
Nursing Clinics of North America		September 2010

15. Extent and Nature of Circulation		Average No. Copies Each Issue During Preceding 12 Months	No. Copies of Single Issue Published Nearest to Filing Date
a. Total Number of Copies (*Net press run*)		2443	2348
b. Paid Circulation (By Mail and Outside the Mail)	(1) Mailed Outside-County Paid Subscriptions Stated on PS Form 3541. (*Include paid distribution above nominal rate, advertiser's proof copies, and exchange copies*)	1463	1458
	(2) Mailed In-County Paid Subscriptions Stated on PS Form 3541 (*Include paid distribution above nominal rate, advertiser's proof copies, and exchange copies*)		
	(3) Paid Distribution Outside the Mails Including Sales Through Dealers and Carriers, Street Vendors, Counter Sales, and Other Paid Distribution Outside USPS®	385	417
	(4) Paid Distribution by Other Classes Mailed Through the USPS (e.g. First-Class Mail®)		
c. Total Paid Distribution (*Sum of 15b (1), (2), (3), and (4)*)	▲	1848	1875
d. Free or Nominal Rate Distribution (By Mail and Outside the Mail)	(1) Free or Nominal Rate Outside-County Copies Included on PS Form 3541	69	63
	(2) Free or Nominal Rate In-County Copies Included on PS Form 3541		
	(3) Free or Nominal Rate Copies Mailed at Other Classes Through the USPS (e.g. First-Class Mail)		
	(4) Free or Nominal Rate Distribution Outside the Mail (Carriers or other means)		
e. Total Free or Nominal Rate Distribution (*Sum of 15d (1), (2), (3) and (4)*)	▲	69	63
f. Total Distribution (*Sum of 15c and 15e*)	▲	1917	1938
g. Copies not Distributed (*See instructions to publishers #4 (page #3)*)	▲	526	410
h. Total (*Sum of 15f and g*)	▲	2443	2348
i. Percent Paid (15c divided by 15f times 100)		96.40%	96.75%

16. Publication of Statement of Ownership

If the publication is a general publication, publication of this statement is required. Will be printed in the **December 2010** issue of this publication. ☐ Publication not required

17. Signature and Title of Editor, Publisher, Business Manager, or Owner

Stephen R. Bushing

Stephen R. Bushing – Fulfillment/Inventory Specialist

Date
September 15, 2010

I certify that all information furnished on this form is true and complete. I understand that anyone who furnishes false or misleading information on this form or who omits material or information requested on the form may be subject to criminal sanctions (including fines and imprisonment) and/or civil sanctions (including civil penalties).

PS Form 3526, September 200 (Page 2 of 3)

Moving?

Make sure your subscription moves with you!

To notify us of your new address, find your **Clinics Account Number** (located on your mailing label above your name), and contact customer service at:

Email: journalscustomerservice-usa@elsevier.com

800-654-2452 (subscribers in the U.S. & Canada)
314-447-8871 (subscribers outside of the U.S. & Canada)

Fax number: 314-447-8029

Elsevier Health Sciences Division
Subscription Customer Service
3251 Riverport Lane
Maryland Heights, MO 63043

*To ensure uninterrupted delivery of your subscription, please notify us at least 4 weeks in advance of move.

Printed and bound by CPI Group (UK) Ltd, Croydon, CR0 4YY

03/10/2024

01040447-0016